SAFE,
WANTED,
AND
LOVED

SAFE,
WANTED,
AND
LOVED

A FAMILY MEMOIR OF
MENTAL ILLNESS,
HEARTBREAK, AND HOPE

PATRICK
DYLAN

SNOW
ANSELMO
PRESS

Published by Snow Anselmo Press, Florida
www.safewantedloved.com

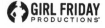

Edited and designed by Girl Friday Productions
www.girlfridayproductions.com

Design: Paul Barrett
Project management: Katherine Richards and Laura Dailey

ISBN (hardcover): 978-1-7364172-2-5
ISBN (paperback): 978-1-7364172-1-8
ISBN (ebook): 978-1-7364172-0-1

Library of Congress Control Number: 2021902606

First edition

For my wife

CONTENTS

That's the stigma. We are so, so, so accepting of any body part breaking down other than our brains. And that's ignorance. That's pure ignorance.

—Kevin Breel, *Confessions of a Depressed Comic*

1.

THE START

Coldplay
"The Scientist"
3:11–3:43

"Pat, I am going to prison."

My wife's voice woke me from a deep sleep. I opened my eyes. The room was dark; it was too early for her to be awake.

I lay still for a few seconds, listening intently. The eeriness of complete silence began to scare me.

"I am going to prison. I am definitely going to prison."

We were staying in the guest room of my parents' house, and being so close in the small bed made Mia's upright posture more apparent.

"What are you talking about, babe?" I asked, trying to sound calm but feeling my pulse quicken. "What time is it?"

"I don't know. That doesn't matter. I am going to be arrested."

The certainty of her answer sent my mind reeling. Mia and I had been together for over seventeen years and married for fourteen. She was as straitlaced and by the book as anyone I had ever met. Sure, she had been pulled over for speeding, but the thought of her doing something that would send her to prison was incomprehensible.

"Mia, you are starting to scare me. What are you talking about?" Her voice sounded different than usual. It was strained and serious. She wasn't joking.

"A family came in to see me on Friday. The boy was severely constipated. I told them to change his diet, but I could have done more. I could have prescribed him a stool softener, but I didn't."

Mia worked as a physician assistant for a highly regarded pediatric firm in our hometown of Sarasota, Florida. She had been in practice for over a decade and was trusted by everyone at her work. I had no medical experience, but what she was saying didn't sound right.

"What? You can't go to prison for that. You did what you thought was best."

She continued as if she couldn't hear me. "It all makes sense now. That family was hired by the doctors to see what my response would be. They must have put a secret camera in the exam room to videotape the whole thing. There must have been several cameras. Oh my God, it's all on tape!"

Now my heart was racing. I couldn't figure out what she was talking about, but she was clearly in distress. And she was wide-awake, as if she hadn't slept at all.

"Calm down, Mia," I said. "I'm sure that your doctors didn't frame you. You did what you thought was best. No one can send you to prison for that. That's just . . . Well, it's crazy."

She sat with her back against the wall, staring into the darkness. In all our time together, I had never seen her look like this. She was clearly worried, but she also appeared deep in thought. She looked like she was analyzing a problem from a thousand angles. Her eyes were glazed over, but she wasn't crying. Although she was talking to me, I wasn't sure if she knew I was there.

Mia and I had met as undergraduates at Harvard. She was extremely intelligent. It was one of the things that I found most attractive about her. Mia wasn't just smart, though, she was creative. She had this incredible gift of looking at the world both in the same way that I did but also in ways that I had never considered.

Another reason I fell in love with Mia was her incredible compassion. People could sense immediately that she truly cared about them and what they were saying. She didn't pretend to hear you; she listened. She didn't feign interest; she really wanted to help.

Mia's kindness didn't mean that she lacked toughness. On the contrary, she was resilient. We met on the track team. She was a highly recruited long-distance runner, nationally ranked and invited to attend every elite university in the country. You don't string together five-minute miles without having serious determination and grit.

I got accepted to Harvard because I had a knack for pole vaulting. Vaulters are good athletes, usually fast and strong, but they aren't known for their determination and grit. Little did I know that on this morning, this darkest of mornings, I would be thrust into a struggle that would severely test my determination and demand all the grit I could muster.

2.

THE FIRST DAY

The Beatles
"I'm Looking Through You"
0:07–0:28

I will never forget the first time I caught sight of Mia. I saw her from across the weight room in Harvard's indoor track facility at the beginning of freshman year. She was petite and naturally elegant, with long dark hair that fell below her shoulders. Her slim build and tan skin were complemented by lively brown eyes, outlined by the longest lashes I had ever seen. Her smile captivated me, and I couldn't stop sneaking glances her way. Watching her, I didn't feel like a small-town kid recently transplanted to a big-city college, timid and alone. I felt young and full of hope.

I heard her tell a friend that she was living in a dormitory called Pennypacker. Later that week, I was out on Saturday with my college roommate, George. We were finishing up a late night of party hopping. Tipsy and hungry, he wanted to go for something to eat.

"First, let's take a walk through Pennypacker," I suggested. "There's a really cute girl on the track team who lives there. Maybe we'll run into her."

He thought it was far-fetched, but George was always a good sport. We soon found ourselves wandering the quiet and deserted hallways of the dorm. As we finished walking the last floor, he lost patience.

"Can we go now? I'm starving!" he whined.

"Yeah, I guess so," I sighed.

George let out an enthusiastic cry of victory and immediately bounded to the stairwell and slipped out of sight, whooping and hollering. As I neared the bottom of the stairs, I heard him accosting someone. "Are you going to eat all of that pizza by yourself?"

"Umm," the person responded, "it's for my roommate and me."

"You guys can't eat all of that pizza," declared George. "C'mon, let us come back to your room and share it with you. C'mon, please? *Please!*"

"Okay. I guess you can come back and have a piece of pizza."

I rounded the final staircase, looked onto the scene, and couldn't believe my luck. George was with the very girl whom I wanted to meet!

Mia led us back to her room. Once there, George, animated and loud, focused his attention on her surprised roommate, who wore an increasingly pained expression.

"I can't believe he talked you into this," I said, gesturing toward George but marveling at the collection of thick science books sprawled across Mia's desk. She was clearly spending her Saturday night much differently than we were.

"Aw, I had to take pity on him," she replied, flashing me that intoxicating smile. "You guys didn't look too dangerous. Besides, he seemed pretty desperate. I felt sorry for him."

"Yeah, well, you should be feeling sorry for your roommate," I joked, and we enjoyed a short conversation about the track team. Mia had recently taken a shower, and I found her damp hair and the fresh smell of her shampoo mesmerizing. Finally, when I couldn't put it off any longer, I dragged George away, a tail end of pizza crust dangling from his fingers.

Once we were out of earshot, George said, "Wow, they were fun. Too bad we didn't meet that girl, though."

"George!" I exclaimed. "That was the girl! Mia was the girl!"

"What? Mia was the girl?" He started jumping up and down.

"Yes! George, you're a genius!" I cried, and we nearly skipped all the way back to our room.

***

"Mia, babe, you need to relax," I said, putting my arms around her. Strangely, she didn't return the hug. "How much sleep did you get last night?"

"I don't remember."

It was Sunday morning, and it happened to be her thirty-ninth birthday. We had celebrated the night before with our two children and my parents. Will, our son, was in sixth grade, and Jamie, our daughter, was in fourth. We had a nice dinner but hadn't stayed up late.

"How much do you think you got?"

"I don't know. I called the office a few times but just left messages. No one was there."

Of course no one was there, I thought. *It was the middle of the night on a Saturday.*

Mia had been unusually worried about her work over the past several months. Her pediatric practice was part of a larger network of physicians. The network was being acquired by the local hospital; doctors and surgeons were vying for position and arguing for salary adjustments. As a physician assistant, Mia was not involved in most of these discussions. But being on the fringe meant even less information, and all of the uncertainty had her on edge.

"Okay, Mia, I know that you have been stressed out about work, and it seems like you haven't slept well. But you aren't thinking clearly. You are not going to prison." I tried to sound reassuring but firm. "Why don't you take a shower and then maybe you'll feel better?"

"Yeah, okay. I'll take a shower."

The water turned on. The dim bedroom was partially lit by the white glare leaking from beneath the bathroom door. I sat in a swirl of crumpled sheets, reflecting on the situation. Mia couldn't get arrested for doing her job, but maybe with all of the shifting allegiances in her office she had upset one of the doctors? It was pretty implausible, given how valuable she was to their practice.

And what was with that glazed look in her eyes? She seemed exhausted but simultaneously anxious and hyper-focused. It was unsettling, like she had stayed up all night and then downed an entire pot of coffee. I decided she must have been suffering from a severe state of overtiredness. I had read about navy SEALs who became disoriented and confused during their training regimen. With a shower, some food, and maybe a nap later in the day, she would be feeling better.

A short time later, we gathered at the door to say good-bye to my mom and stepdad. We would be heading home that afternoon after stopping to spend the day with Mia's family in Roseland.

"Thanks for the great birthday dinner," Mia said as she hugged my mom. "I really enjoyed it." My mom, a former runner as well, was also slight and athletic. As she responded, I kept a close eye on my wife. Mia was acting normal, saying all the things that you would expect. She still had an unusual look in her eyes, but the paranoid thoughts seemed to have cleared.

Ever since having children, Mia did most of the driving. She had developed motion sickness, and if she wasn't behind the wheel, she became nauseous. So as usual that morning, Mia took her place in the driver's seat. As we came to a light, I found it odd that she hadn't put on her directional signal. "You're going to turn here, right?"

"Yes, but I'm not going to turn right. It's a left turn," she responded in a flat voice, flicking on her blinker. She hadn't quite understood what I meant.

The entire drive was like that. She stared blankly ahead, and I reminded her of the route. The kids didn't notice anything, sitting behind us in the minivan, but I studied her every move with a growing unease.

We met Mia's family at church for Mass. Her reserved parents, Marcos and Lucia Delgado, were two of the friendliest people I knew. Both small in stature like Mia, they had come to the US during the Cuban Revolution in the early 1960s and worked hard to build a life together, raising four children in a strict Catholic home. Conservative like his parents, her older brother, Mark, was an emergency room doctor. Her younger sister, Celia, was an office manager and the most outspoken of the family. Seven grandkids had graced the family. Mia also had a younger brother, Luke, who was not at the church that morning.

Our large family sat down together along a few pews in the back, and the methodical hour of the service gave me a chance to calm my worries. Yes, my wife had been acting very strange. But she was clearly tired, and people needed their sleep. Once Mia had a chance to rest, everything would be fine.

When church was over, we drove to her sister's place. More extroverted than Mia, Celia had a big heart and an even bigger personality. Whenever the Delgado family gathered, her voice was the loudest of the group, dominating the conversation and carrying across the house. The boys of the family had planned a golf outing, followed by a late lunch at Celia's. The whole day had been scheduled months in advance. I was hesitant to leave Mia, but I didn't want to make a scene.

"How are you feeling, babe?" I asked. "Are you still worried about work?"

"No, I'm fine," she promised. "Go have fun. Everything is okay."

I looked into her eyes but didn't feel like we were connecting. Still, she was saying all the right things, and I knew our son would be disappointed if we didn't play. Will lived for golf and had been excited for weeks. I figured a few hours away wouldn't hurt. Besides, Mia would be with her family.

About forty-five minutes into the round, I overheard my brother-in-law Mark talking on the phone. He was a likable guy, smart and self-confident, but with his shaved head and round John Lennon glasses, he could resemble an imposing professor, especially when things turned serious.

"What? Celia, calm down. Repeat what you just said," he ordered, trying to concentrate. He listened for a while longer and then glanced over at me. He pulled the phone away from his ear. "Was Mia acting weird this morning? Celia is freaking out."

All my concern from the morning came rushing back. "Yeah, she was," I said. "Let me talk to her."

Fortunately, Will and his cousins were off near the green, oblivious to what was happening. "Celia, it's Pat."

"Pat, oh my God, Mia is really starting to scare us!" she pleaded in a terrified voice.

I tried to sound composed. "Celia, calm down. Tell me what's going on."

"It's like she's gone crazy. She says that people at her work are after her, that they've got secret cameras recording her. She says it's all linked to some books that she's been reading to the kids. She keeps saying we have to contact the author of these books because he has the answer. What the hell is she talking about?"

It sounded even worse than before, and I felt a hit of adrenaline. "She was acting strange before church, too. I don't think she slept last night. She just needs some sleep." I said it like I knew what I was talking about.

"Sleep, there's no way she's going to sleep!" cried Celia. "She's wired, and she's scaring me. At first, I thought she was kidding, but she's completely serious. She thinks the cops are after her!" Celia was frantic. "You and Mark need to get back here!"

"Okay," I said, trying to calm myself down, too. "You're right. Just do your best until we get there."

I hung up the phone and looked at Mark, suddenly relieved to have an emergency room doctor in the family.

Although my heart was pounding, I tried to slow my voice and clearly explain to him my interactions with Mia that morning. We had known each other for over fifteen years, but I had never seen Mark in a clinical setting. He immediately started rattling off questions.

"Did you notice anything out of the ordinary before this morning?"

"Not really."

"Do you know how much sleep Mia actually got last night?"

"No."

"Do you know what her sleeping patterns have been like over the past week?"

"No."

"Has she seemed more anxious than usual recently?"

"Yeah, she has been worried about her work."

"Has she complained about headaches more than usual?"

"You know she suffers from migraines, but I haven't noticed anything different."

"Has she been taking any medications or drugs of any kind?"

"No, nothing."

He said he would have to see her to know more. We told the kids that Aunt Mia wasn't feeling well and that we had to go back to check on her.

Will shot me a worried look. He had inherited Mia's dark eyes and long lashes. I knelt down to reassure him, his wavy brown hair framing the concern on his face. He was just beginning to make the transition from child to teenager, and he had always been sensitive. "She's going to be fine," I promised him quietly.

It was a silent ride from the golf course to Celia's place. Mark and I were deliberately not talking about the situation in front of the kids. *She just needs to sleep*, I kept repeating to myself in a state of bewildered shock.

Walking into the house, we saw Mia sitting at the kitchen table with Celia and Mark's wife, Kim. Mark and I went over to join them while my father-in-law, Marcos, took the boys outside to join the other cousins playing in the pool.

"Hi, you guys," Celia said as she saw us come in. "How was golf?" She was speaking like someone overacting in an attempt to sound normal. At any other time, Mia would have immediately noticed, but she only glanced up with a strange smile on her face. I was reminded of a person who has had too many drinks and sits there oblivious to the fact that everyone else knows she is drunk.

"It was fine," said Mark, "really fun. What are you three doing?"

"Oh," said Kim, "we've been spending time on the internet." She was an experienced nurse and, like Mark, more poised than Celia and I. "Mia really wanted to know the details about the author of a book series she has been reading to her kids called The 39 Clues. But it turns out that there are several books in that series, all written by different authors."

"Yes," said Mia, looking at me with that odd smile, "but that's just the cover story. Whoever wrote those books has the answer, I'm sure of it. It's all starting to make sense."

"Yeah," said Celia, "Mia has been saying that a lot, that things are making sense. We've been taking notes, see?"

She handed me a piece of paper that was covered in scribbles. Most of the comments were in Mia's handwriting, but Celia and Kim had added things, too:

The 39 Clues—track down the author and find the answer!—This was double underlined.

Doctors secretive, what are they hiding?—This wasn't surprising, given what was happening at her work.

The bishop knows and must have sent the devil.—This last one was in small print, in Mia's handwriting, and was clearly disturbing.

The whole sheet was covered by paranoid ravings. Mia was saying stuff that made absolutely no sense, but she adamantly believed it. The realization froze me in place as I stared at that damned piece of paper.

"Mia, I know you're concerned about your work," said Mark, gesturing toward the garage. "Why don't you come outside, and we can talk about it?"

"Why would we go to the garage?" asked Mia, puzzled at the odd request.

"I want to get some air," replied Mark. "Besides, it's nice out."

His last comment was ridiculous. It was September in South Florida. The temperature was about a million degrees with high humidity. But Mia didn't ask any more questions; she followed Mark out the door. Celia turned to me.

"Holy shit!" She couldn't hold it together anymore. "What the hell's going on? Mia has gone crazy! You heard her. You saw her. It's not normal!"

I felt darkness creeping in from all sides, like a nightmare where you sense a menacing presence in the space around you. Mia was so smart, her thoughts always so rational. *This cannot be happening,* I told myself, unable to tear my eyes from the page of demented notes.

"Did you hear me?" demanded Celia. "She's been this way since we got here, talking about the people at her work being after her, and all of this crazy shit about the clues and the answer! Are you listening to me? Pat!"

Her shout jerked me back to reality, and I looked up from the paper. "I know, I know, it doesn't make sense," I said, my voice cracking. "Everything seemed fine last night, but when she woke up, she kept saying she was going to prison."

"Yeah, no kidding. We just heard that about a hundred times!"

"I know, but she seemed fine after church. She was acting normal again. I'm telling you, she just needs to get some sleep."

"Sleep! Can someone go crazy just because they haven't slept at night?" asked Celia. "No, I'm not buying that! We used to pull all-nighters in college."

"I'm not saying this is from missing one night of sleep. She's been worried for weeks. She might not have slept for days."

"But that's not normal, Pat. When people get tired, they sleep. They don't go crazy!"

"But people don't just go crazy, Celia," I countered. "What are you saying, that Mia has somehow come down with a case of schizophrenia?"

"I don't know. I'm just so worried about her!"

"I'm worried, too," I replied, my tone softening.

"Mark will figure it out," interjected Kim.

As if on cue, Mark poked his head through the garage door. "Hey, Pat, why don't you come out and join us?" he asked, his eyebrows drawn together in a solemn expression. It must have been how he appeared in the emergency room.

Stepping into the garage was like walking into a sauna. Rather than keep her car in there, Celia used the space for extra storage. All kinds of bikes, balls, and skateboards covered the floor and various shelves.

"Mia is really worried about work," Mark said. "I was thinking maybe the two of you could take a walk and talk about it. She always feels more comfortable with you around."

"Okay, sure," I said, smiling uncomfortably. I could feel my blood pumping fast as I took Mia's hand, leading her out of the garage and into the baking sunshine. She continued prattling on about work and clues and hidden messages. We meandered a couple of driveways down the street, but it was way too hot to be outside. I directed us back to Celia's garage to get out of the sun. Mark had returned inside the house.

It was unsettling, to be walking so closely with the person I loved and to be so unnerved. I didn't know how to act. Should I play along with her crazy rants, would that reinforce her behavior? Should I try to reason with her, even though that seemed pointless?

As we walked into the garage, Mia became more agitated. She was explaining to me about her work, and how they had started hiding cameras around the office weeks and probably months ago. Somehow this was connected to a secret clue hidden in these books that she had been reading to the kids.

"We need to figure out where the author lives, Pat!" she pleaded. She continued holding my hand, imploring me as if her demand were somehow rational. "He can tell us why this is happening. He can tell us why it all started!"

She stopped abruptly, and her face went pale. "Oh my God, we need to go back to the beginning! We need to go in reverse!"

Her eyes widened, terror shining through them. "We need to go back!" she screeched.

"Mia, listen to me," I said, trying to hold her close. I was using as comforting a voice as I could manage. "You need to relax. You just need to get some sleep."

"Sleep? What do you mean, 'sleep'?" she gasped, squirming out of my embrace.

"Well, I'm not sure that you slept last night."

"What! What are you talking about? I didn't sleep last night?" she asked, her voice loud and demanding.

"Babe, I don't think so. Do you know if you did?"

"OH MY GOD, I DIDN'T SLEEP LAST NIGHT!!"

"Calm down, don't shout," I said. I was concerned that the kids would hear her yelling.

"Why not!?" she asked. "Something is really wrong, Pat! Something is really wrong!" She started screaming,

"Oh my God, I didn't sleep! We need to go back to the beginning! WE NEED TO GO BACK!!"

I stood immobile, thunderstruck. My wife, whom I had never heard yell in my life, was shrieking nonsense to me at the top of her lungs.

"It's The 39 Clues!" she cried. "You need to listen to me, Pat! We need to go back! We need to reverse everything! OH MY GOD!! OH MY GOD!!"

And then she just started screaming louder than I thought possible.

Mark saved me again. He came rushing out to the garage.

"Hey, Mia, what's all the shouting about?" he asked in a harsh voice, louder than usual to be heard over Mia's screams. She stopped yelling and turned frantically toward him. Kim had come into the garage, too.

"Keep quiet," Mark ordered. "We're going back to our house now. We know you have a lot to talk about, and we're going someplace private so the four of us can figure this out."

"Yes!" cried Mia. "We need to figure this out. It's all got to mean something." She remained hysterical, but she had stopped screaming.

"Oh absolutely," agreed Mark emphatically. "I absolutely think that this means something. And we're going to find out what."

He turned and gave Kim a quick nod. She strode forward, took Mia's arm, and started walking her to the driveway. At the same time, Mark pulled me aside.

"Pat, Mia is suffering from acute psychosis. That means that her brain is not functioning properly. Her thoughts are not based in reality. I have seen this before in the emergency room." He was speaking quickly without showing the type of panic that I was feeling. He stopped, and his voice softened. "Dude, I know, it's scary."

Mark immediately became the expert again. "We need to get her to the emergency room, but we have to do it in the right way. We are going to get her out of here, away from the kids, and then I'll need some time to arrange things. Just go with it for now. We'll talk in detail later." He had led me to his truck. I climbed into the back seat, next to Mia.

I sat in stunned silence as Mark drove, adrenaline coursing through my body. For over twenty-one years—as long as I had known her—the thought of being next to Mia was so comforting; but, sitting beside her in that truck, it felt like standing in front of a firing line, bracing for the first shot.

Mark and Kim maintained a continuous dialogue with Mia during the trip. She seemed to gain comfort by talking and having people answer without telling her to calm down. Their conversation would have sounded deranged to any eavesdropper.

"So, this author has the answer?" Mark asked.

"Yeah, he has the answer. It's somewhere in those books."

"And the doctors have been working on something without telling you?" Kim followed up.

"Yes, they have been. They've been videotaping the rooms, too. I think they've been tapping the phones."

Their exchange gave me the opportunity to digest what was happening. Back in college I had taken a psychology class, and I had read about mental health disorders. I knew that the brain functioned with the help of various chemicals, and that these chemicals interacted with neurons. But I had never been around anyone with a serious mental illness. I had certainly never interacted with someone who was psychotic.

In my head, I began formulating an explanation for Mia's startling behavior. Anxiety surrounding the upcoming changes at work had affected her sleeping patterns. She had reached a state of overtiredness that had somehow become unstable. The stress and lack of sleep had thrown the chemical balance in her brain completely out of whack.

Mark seemed to have been thinking the same thing. "So, Mia, when we get to our house, what do you think about trying to take a nap?"

"I'm not tired."

"Yes, but you were up early," said Kim. "Let's just lie down for a while, and then we'll be ready to talk about everything."

By the time we arrived, Mark and Kim had somehow talked Mia into trying to take a nap. Kim took her into their bedroom, and I stayed with Mark in the living room.

"Okay, like I said, we need to get Mia to the emergency room," he said.

"Really? You don't think she'll be better once she gets some sleep?"

Mark furrowed his brow and frowned. "She's not going to sleep," he said matter-of-factly. "Pat, let me make something clear to you. This is a serious medical situation. Acute psychosis isn't something to toy with. It could have an organic cause. If it does, we need to know immediately."

I was startled by his grave tone and offended that he thought I was taking it lightly. "I know this is serious, Mark, but speak English. I don't know what you just said."

"Look, Mia's brain is not working. We need to find out why. It could be a brain tumor; I don't know. It could be a number of things. We need to run tests, lots of them."

I hadn't considered a brain tumor. The only thing worse than Mia in her current state would be Mia with some type of terminal disease, something that couldn't be treated. My face must have reflected my thoughts, and Mark quickly added, "I'm not telling you that Mia has brain cancer, but we need to know what we're dealing with."

"Okay, let's get her to the hospital."

"It's not that easy," he said. "If we Baker Act her, we'll lose all control over the situation. Plus, it will probably keep her from getting a job in the future."

"What are you talking about? What is Baker Acting?" I hated the sound of it.

"Sorry. Baker Acting means committing someone to a mental health facility against their will. We can't make Mia go to the hospital, and she might not want to go. You saw how she started screaming back there in Celia's garage. If we call 911, they will take her away to the closest facility and put her in lockdown."

"Good Lord," I gasped, "are they allowed to do that? Just take her away from us like that?"

"A hundred percent they can do that, especially if they think she might hurt herself or someone else."

"Mia would never hurt anyone! You know that, Mark."

"I'm not saying she would, but people with psychosis are unpredictable. Mia can't control her thoughts. Basically, right now *that*"—he pointed to the bedroom—"is not Mia."

That was a sickening concept, but it made the situation a bit easier to comprehend. "Okay, so what do we do?"

He said he was going to call his cousin Alex. In the commotion of the day, I had forgotten that Mia's cousin was a psychiatrist. He ran a successful practice down in Miami; I knew him from family holidays. Mark pulled out his cell phone and dialed the number.

"Alex, yeah, it's me. We have a real problem here. Mia woke up psychotic. Yes, mostly paranoid. I don't know. No, no prior signs, but it seems to be progressing." As Mark started talking, it felt like a movie; it couldn't be my life.

"I need to get her to the emergency room. I know, but I can't Baker Act her. I can't do that to my sister. No, I know, Alex, but I'm not going to do that!" Obviously, Alex's professional opinion was to send Mia to a mental health facility.

"Right, I could do that. I do know someone with an affiliation. Yes, she'll have to agree to go on her own. I know, that's what I'm concerned about." Mark glanced my way. "Yeah, he'll have to. It's the only way. Okay, thanks. I'll keep you updated." Mark hung up the phone and stood staring at me.

"What's the plan?" I asked.

"Okay, you have to know this, Pat. Those crisis units at the mental health facility—they are the most depressing places you can imagine. I can't put Mia in there. I just can't do it to her."

"Fine!" I almost screamed. "I don't want to do that, either. What's the other option?"

"I'll call the emergency room and get things prepared. We'll get Mia admitted to the hospital, and we'll order a ton of tests. I know a psychiatrist who can see her there. And we'll get some sedatives in her so she can sleep."

"That's perfect!" I said, feeling that my prayers had been answered. "What do you want me to do?"

"That's the key to all this. You have to convince her to go. You know how paranoid she is right now. We can't force her into the hospital, so it's up to you. If she refuses to get admitted, the whole thing will fall apart. Then, we won't have a choice. We'll have to Baker Act her."

I felt an incredible surge of energy. In a surreal day filled with so much fear and confusion, I finally knew what I had to do.

"Leave it to me," I said, suddenly confident. "Let's go save Mia."

3.

THE EMERGENCY ROOM

Pearl Jam
"Black"
0:49–1:10

After meeting in her dorm over pizza, Mia and I dated for a couple of weeks, but then she broke it off. She was sweet about it, using the excuse that she needed to concentrate on her studies. It was disappointing but not unexpected; Mia was way more academically focused than I was.

Three months later and home for the holidays, I received a letter from her. Surprised, I opened it to find a delicate card with the image of a dove and the word *Peace* outlined in gold against a white background. Inside, Mia had written:

Pat, Merry Christmas! I really enjoyed meeting you this fall. Even though we broke up, I truly hope that we can remain friends. Love, Mia

Given Mia's personality, it was impossible not to remain her friend. In the years that followed, we met every month or two for lunch and saw each other randomly at social events.

By the spring of our senior year, we were basically done with graduation requirements. One night, I ran into Mia at a house party. At Harvard, a house is a blend of apartment building, dormitory, and social community. After their first year, students are sorted into one of a dozen houses, and it becomes their home during the rest of their time on campus.

Mia lived in Dunster House, which was far from the party at Cabot House where we met that night. But hers was the first face I noticed across the crowded room, and we had a great time hanging out together. A few days later, she called me unexpectedly. She wanted to know if I was attending my house formal, an elegant dance that each house held at the end of the semester.

"Nah, I'm not going."

"What? You aren't going to your last formal?" She sounded appalled.

"I don't have anyone to go with," I replied, a broad grin stretching across my face.

"Oh, come on, I'll go with you."

She had basically invited herself to my house formal, but I still assumed it was strictly platonic.

A large group of us met at a restaurant before the event. Mia and I were sitting at one end of a long table, next to my roommate, George, the same guy from the pizza incident. It was a fancy place, with way too many extra forks and spoons. Given that we were all poor students, a heavy awkwardness descended as we studied the prices.

"So, what's it gonna be, bub?" quipped Mia, peering across her oversize menu at me with a sarcastic grin. Her comment sliced right through the pretension; George and I loved it. The chemistry was special that night, and the three of us laughed our way through dinner.

Later, during the dance, George pulled me aside. "I never knew Mia was so funny! She's awesome."

"I know," I agreed, watching Mia from across the room. He followed my gaze and knew what I was thinking.

"Yeah," he chuckled, slapping me on the back, "too bad she dumped you!" He gave a snort and walked away.

He's right, I thought. *I shouldn't let myself daydream.*

And I didn't, until the end of the evening. Mia surprised me with a kiss.

"I had a great time tonight, Pat," she confessed, treating me to an up-close view of those captivating eyes. "How about giving things another try?"

She didn't need to say it twice.

***

I slowly opened the door to Mark and Kim's bedroom. The room was dark, almost like nighttime. Mark's hours in the emergency room could be rough, and he had installed blackout curtains so he could sleep during the day. Kim heard me come in.

"I was just about to come and get you," she whispered. "Mia isn't asleep, but we were talking quietly. Go ahead and take my place."

As Kim left the room, I lay down next to Mia.

"I'm glad you're here," she said so softly, and with so much feeling, that I suddenly thought the psychosis had cleared. "Kim is acting weird."

"What do you mean, 'acting weird'?"

"Look at this. It's the middle of the day, and we're lying here in the dark."

Mia was right; it was strange to be lying in total darkness when it was so bright outside. Maybe lying down had brought her thoughts back into focus. "So, how are you doing? You were a little upset earlier, but now you seem better."

"I'm okay. I'm trying to figure out why everyone is acting so weird. What are we doing in bed? We need to start figuring things out."

I lost hope at this last comment. Somehow, I had to persuade her to go to the emergency room. That seemed impossible at the moment.

"You may not remember, but you woke up really early this morning," I said. "So, Mark thought you might want to take a nap. Plus, I woke up early with you, and I'm pretty tired."

"I didn't realize that you were tired."

"Yeah, well, we both got up at 5:30 a.m."

"I'm sorry." Even in her current state, Mia's inherent compassion came through. "I'll be quiet," she said, "and maybe you can rest."

I had never been able to nap during the day. Mia, on the other hand, had always fallen asleep almost immediately. At any other time, I would have heard her breathing slow within ten minutes, and then she would have started twitching.

But that didn't happen. As time dragged on, I found myself becoming increasingly anxious. We had to get Mia to the hospital, and I was wasting time. I could feel her thoughts racing furiously beside me in the distressing silence. After what seemed like a half hour, I couldn't stand it anymore.

"You're not asleep, are you?" I whispered.

"No," she whispered back.

"Isn't that strange?" I asked. "I mean, when else over the past twenty years have you not fallen asleep within five minutes of lying down?"

"Yeah, I guess. I was too busy thinking about work."

"Look, babe," I said. "Mark told me that sometimes people get overtired. It especially happens when they are thinking about work a lot. He suggested that if you couldn't fall asleep, we might want to get something to help you." I knew that she respected Mark's opinion as much as I did.

"You mean like lorazepam?" she asked. This was typical of Mia; whenever the conversation turned to anything medical, I was quickly in over my head. I decided to wing it.

"Yeah, something like that," I replied, hoping it wouldn't get me into trouble. I had no idea what *lorazepam* was.

"That might help me relax. Would he call it out?" I realized that she had asked if Mark was going to call the pharmacy with a prescription.

"No, not exactly," I said. "He thought it would be best to go over to the hospital. Given that he works in the emergency room, he said it would be faster. Plus, they'd be sure to have whatever we need." I hoped it sounded believable.

"Really? That's odd. Why would he say that?"

I started to panic. Of course, she was right. Mark would never have suggested that. No wonder she thought everyone was acting weird—we *were* acting weird. I was trying to formulate some plausible reason why I had suggested this, when Mia spoke again.

"Maybe the pharmacies around here aren't reliable," she said. "Maybe they don't carry even the most basic prescriptions."

She hadn't been addressing me when she posed the question. She had been talking to herself, and she had devised a rationale that would never have crossed my mind.

"That's probably it," I agreed quickly.

"But to go all the way to the hospital for something like lorazepam? That doesn't seem right."

"Well, that's what Mark said. When it comes to that kind of thing, he knows what he's talking about."

"But it's not like he can prescribe anything for me in the hospital. He's my brother; I can't be his patient."

I hadn't considered this, but she was right again. I said the first thing that came to mind. "He said he knows the doctor working right now, so it wouldn't be an issue. He said it'd be really easy this way."

"Really easy to get me prescriptions . . . easier than calling it out . . ." She was still talking to herself, and something told me to remain silent. I couldn't think of anything to say anyway.

"Okay," she said, sounding tentative.

"Great," I responded quickly. "Well, obviously we're not going to fall asleep here. Let's go tell Mark that we should head over to the hospital."

We were soon back in his truck, where the conversation returned to the bizarre. Mia was focused on religion, explaining that the devil was real. She thought Satan must have something to do with the current situation—the clues and her work and everything.

"I bet our local bishop summoned the devil before we left and told him to follow us," she concluded. "He must have been hiding in our trunk on the drive over here. I wonder if he's still in there or if he escaped over at Celia's house."

This didn't sound anything like the Mia I had married, but I was only partially listening. Mostly, I was willing the truck to go faster.

Mark's hospital was in Melbourne, a half hour away. The drive was painfully long, but upon arrival we were swept into the mayhem of the emergency room. Mark led Mia through a door at the back while I checked her in. It took time to answer all the admitting questions and provide insurance information. When the process was over, I found myself in a hallway with Mark. He was introducing me to Dr. Adams, the physician on duty. She was young and smart looking.

"Hi, Pat. I know you and Mia have had a tough day," said the doctor, who had a friendly disposition. "We're going to see if we can get her to relax a bit. She's a little agitated, so maybe you can help her calm down until the medication takes effect?"

As she said this, she opened the door to a room. I saw Mia lying on one of those movable hospital beds, her small body surrounded by a large mattress that was propped up in the back. A nurse was circling around. The obligatory blood pressure machine was close by, and Mia already had an IV in her arm. She looked up as I entered.

"Pat!" she blurted out, surprised to see me. "Where did you go? This is overkill, look at all this!"

"Um," I stammered, "well, I guess they have their procedures."

"Procedures? No, this isn't right. Let's get Mark and tell him to get us out of here."

I noticed that Mark and Dr. Adams had remained in the hallway. "It does seem kind of over the top," I agreed, "but we've come all this way. Let's stay a little longer."

At that moment, the nurse approached with a syringe. "Mia, the doctor thought this would help you relax. It's Ativan, and I'm just going to put it through your IV."

"Right, lorazepam," said Mia. I would soon become quite familiar with Ativan, or its generic name, lorazepam. It was a sedative regularly used to treat anxiety. Lorazepam wouldn't necessarily put you to sleep, but it would sedate you. It would also wreak havoc with your short-term memory, but I hadn't learned about that side effect yet.

"What about you, Pat?" Mia asked. "You were having trouble sleeping today. We should probably start these *procedures* for you." She said the last comment aggressively.

Then the nurse, who had finished with the sedative, started asking questions. "So, Mia, I understand that you haven't had a lot of sleep lately?"

"I guess not." She stared crossly at me as she said it.

"And you've been under a lot of stress at work?" The nurse was trying to be nice, but he was fighting a losing battle.

"Yes, I have." Even though Mia was curt and unhappy, I was amazed by how normal she was acting. I held my breath, waiting for the paranoid thoughts to start spilling out.

"Okay." The nurse paused. "Can you tell me, are you currently taking any medications?"

"No."

"Do you use alcohol or recreational drugs?"

Mia gave me that look again. She was losing patience fast. "No, I don't. How many questions do you have?"

At this point, Dr. Adams came in. "Hello again, Mia," she said. "I see that you have been reunited with your husband. How are you feeling now? Do you feel more comfortable?" She was trying to determine if the Ativan had started working.

"Yes, I do. I feel much better. Thank you." Mia had never been a good liar. "It is probably time for us to go."

The doctor ignored her, turning to me. "We've given her a sedative, which should help her relax."

Dr. Adams looked back toward Mia. "Don't worry, we won't keep you here long. I'm just going to ask you a few more questions. Now, do you have any family history of depression?"

Mia had, in fact, suffered postpartum blues following the birth of Will. As she was telling the doctor this, Mark entered the room, tugged my shoulder, and motioned toward the door. I hesitated and then followed.

"Mark, I think I better stay in there. She's getting pretty upset," I said as the door closed behind us.

"It's okay. The sedative should kick in soon." He gave a terse shake of his head, indicating that Mia's anger didn't concern him. "I wanted to let you know what we're planning. We'll be running all kinds of blood tests to see if anything is going on organically. Some of those will take a while to get back. We'll also be doing an EKG, an EEG, and a CT scan of her brain."

"Wow, okay," I said, remembering the brain tumor conversation and then trying to forget it. "How long will all that stuff take? She doesn't want to stick around."

"She won't be leaving tonight, Pat. I don't want you leaving, either. We'll admit her to the hospital, and you can sleep in her room." His voice was a mix of clinician and compassionate brother-in-law. I realized that Mark was worried; he thought we would find something in one of the tests.

"What about the kids?" I asked. They both had school the next morning, and we still had to make the three-hour drive home to Sarasota. "Jesus, what time is it?"

"It's just before six. Don't worry about the kids. My mom and dad are taking care of them. They'll miss a day of school, but that's the least of our concerns right now."

"I should probably call them." I started to reach for the phone in my pocket. Mark stopped me.

"It won't be much longer, and then you can call. I want to be sure Mia calms down so that we can start the tests." He opened the door, and I took that as my cue to return to her side. She was still answering questions.

"No, I don't remember," she was saying. She turned to Mark and me. "Can we leave now?" she asked, but she didn't seem as angry.

"No, not yet. I'd like to run some tests, just to rule out any other reasons for your unusual sleeping patterns over the past few days," said Dr. Adams.

Mia frowned, but when she spoke, her voice had lost its edge. "When will that happen?"

"We'll do it now," replied Mark, sensing the change in Mia's mood. "It won't take long." He turned to me. "Pat, I'll stay with her during these tests. You can just hang out in the waiting area."

"Okay," I said, turning to Mia. "I love you, babe. I'll be right here when the tests are over." I leaned over to give her a kiss, but she ignored me. I left the room as the nurse was busy preparing what looked like vials for taking blood.

I walked to the waiting room and then kept going. I thought my phone would get better coverage outside, plus I needed fresh air. A weight was lifted off my shoulders, and I realized it was the stress of being around Mia. It felt like carrying around a stick of dynamite.

Releasing the tension in my back, I took a deep breath and called the cell number for my mother-in-law, Lucia. She answered, and I provided a brief update. She was quiet and supportive, and then she put the kids on the phone.

I spoke first to Jamie, who answered in her typically upbeat way. I could picture her sandy-brown hair tied back in a ponytail as she probably half listened to me and half concentrated on a picture she was drawing. Jamie was always doing something creative.

"When will we be going home, Daddy?" she asked, hiding any concern that she might be feeling about Mia's health. I told her it would be soon and that everything would be okay. She seemed satisfied with that.

Will wasn't so easy. I told him the same thing, but, from his mumbled responses and silent pauses, I could tell that he wasn't buying it.

Next, I called my mom. I wanted to see if she had noticed anything unusual about Mia's behavior that morning or over the weekend. It sounded strange telling my mom that Mia was psychotic. The word had been poisoned by pop culture. I phrased it as "Mia is suffering from psychosis," which sounded more acceptable.

"Oh, honey, I'm so sorry," my mom said, her familiar and sympathetic voice lending me strength. "You know, Mia did seem more reserved than usual . . . quiet, like something was on her mind. But no, nothing like what you are describing."

She wanted to know what was causing the strange behavior, but I didn't have an answer. I realized how much I didn't know about the brain.

Returning to the waiting room, I opened the browser on my phone and googled *acute psychosis*. This brought up all kinds of links to schizophrenia-related articles. I wasn't ready to contemplate something as serious as that. Instead, I went to the *psychosis* entry on Wikipedia. It talked about a "loss of contact with reality," which certainly sounded like Mia's situation. It also described various impairments associated with psychosis. She didn't suffer from hallucinations, like hearing voices and seeing things, or from catatonia, moving in an uncontrolled way.

But the article also mentioned delusions—false beliefs that a person clung to without adequate evidence. It said that oftentimes these could be paranoid in nature. That was a clear yes in Mia's case. The other impairment was thought disorder, which referred to people misinterpreting what they heard or read. I remembered how Mia misunderstood certain things I was saying, like how she mistook "you're going to turn here, right?" for "you're going to turn right here."

Reading about psychosis made me feel a little better. At least, it confirmed that this had happened to other people. But my heart sank as I reviewed the possible causes. Dozens of reasons were listed, and many sounded bad. Brain issues, like tumors, were prevalent. Articles also mentioned diseases of the endocrine system, mostly dealing with the thyroid.

Outside of these "organic" causes, dozens of mental health disorders were described. They all sounded scary, too. I read that bipolar disorder involved periods of both depression and mania, and that someone going through a manic phase could become psychotic.

I was still lost in research when Mark returned to the waiting room. I had been reading for over an hour, alone among a small collection of tattered chairs and side tables. Most of what I learned only increased my concern, especially the part about brain cancer, and he could sense my apprehension.

"The CT scan was normal," he said quickly. "She doesn't have any sign of a tumor."

"Oh, thank God." Relief washed over me.

"Yeah, that's the good news," he said. "The bad news is that we still don't know what's going on. But I'll admit, Pat, I was worried. If we had found a tumor, it would have been terrible. Then it's the kids grow up without a mommy."

"Let's not think about that now," I said, changing the subject. "Where do we go from here?"

"We can make our way back to the ER. She'll have a break before the next round of tests."

Mia was in the same room where we had left her, lying on the oversize bed, her dark hair spilling across the white pillow. "Hello again, Pat," said Dr. Adams, who was standing nearby. "Mia and I were just talking. I thought she'd be feeling comfortable by now, but she still seems a bit tense."

"I feel okay," said Mia, looking up at us, "but it's time to leave."

Dr. Adams glanced down at Mia. "Your wife can be pretty stubborn."

"Yeah, I learned that a long time ago." I smiled at Mia. She was clearly not as aggressive as before, but she didn't seem on the threshold of sleep, either. I took her hand. "Still not feeling tired, babe?"

Before Mia could answer, Mark spoke up. "Hey, guys, I'm going to the office with Dr. Adams. Pat, why don't you stay here with Mia? We'll be back soon."

On their way out, Mark turned down the lights. We were left in the dimly lit room, with only beeps from the various machines to break the silence. My anxiety began to build again, as I waited, alone in Mia's presence.

"How long do we have to stay here?" Mia asked. She was looking at me, but it was a blank stare.

"Mark wants us to spend the night," I replied. "He wants to make sure you get some sleep."

"I don't want to stay here," she said. "I'll sleep at home. We still have to drive home." Suddenly, her eyes grew wide and she looked frightened. "We have to get the kids home, Pat! Where are the kids?"

"The kids are fine," I said, stroking her arm. I knew from experience that a light stroke on Mia's arm could calm her anxiety. "I just talked to them. They're safe and sound at your parents' house. Mark wants us both to sleep here tonight."

I held my breath, but the strategy worked. Mia relaxed and glanced across the room. After a moment she sighed and muttered, "This is so weird. Why is everyone acting so weird?" She seemed to be talking to herself again, so I let the question linger.

Mia was slowly scanning the room; I could tell that her brain didn't want to slow down. I wondered what she was thinking, but I also wondered how much medication she could tolerate before giving up. Not much had changed when the doctors returned a short while later.

"How are we doing?" inquired Dr. Adams.

"About the same," I replied. "We're still pretty awake in here."

"Looks that way," said Mark. "Pat, you need dinner. I'll show you to the cafeteria. Dr. Adams is going to coordinate a few more tests."

"Oh, you haven't eaten," said Mia. "You should get some dinner." Apparently, the fact that she, too, hadn't eaten anything since breakfast failed to register.

"Okay," I said hesitantly, looking from Mia to Mark and back again. I stood up and kissed Mia on the cheek. "I'll be back soon, babe."

I felt an uncomfortable mix of relief and then guilt upon leaving the room. Mark ushered me through byzantine corridors as we made our way to the cafeteria. He was busy informing me about the tests they had completed and those they were planning.

So far, Mia had received only a small dose of Ativan. They were waiting to use more until all the tests had been run. Other medications would definitely put her to sleep, but they didn't want to use them until she had been seen by a psychiatrist. Only a specialist could determine the best drug to combat her psychosis. Mark called these antipsychotic medications "hardcore psychotropic drugs." I would soon learn much about them.

The eating area was sterile and bleak, with several blurry-eyed workers huddled in scrubs and engaged in quiet conversation. Mark and I talked while we ate, discussing possible reasons for Mia's disconcerting behavior. Mostly this meant Mark throwing out potential causes and trying to describe complicated medical conditions to someone without adequate training. I followed some of his explanations but got lost in others.

After twenty minutes, Mark received a text. He looked up from his phone. "The other tests are done, and Dr. Patel is on his way. He's a psychiatrist I know with admitting privileges here. He can prescribe the antipsychotic."

"He can give Mia the sleeping medication?" I asked.

"Yeah, that's the plan."

"Great, let's get back there," I said, still believing that she would be okay after getting some sleep. Anything else to me was unfathomable.

4.

THE FIRST DIAGNOSIS

Bruce Springsteen
"Waitin' on a Sunny Day"
2:38–3:11

Although Mia and I were inseparable during the last month of college, we didn't expect our relationship to last past graduation. I had already committed to an investment banking job in Chicago. Beginning in July, I would be working eighty hours a week in a high-rise near the Board of Trade. I wasn't thrilled about it, but I was deep in student debt and needed the money.

Mia was in the process of determining her next move, but Chicago wasn't in her plans. I always thought she would become a doctor, but as we spent time together, it became clear that she was giving more careful thought to her career.

"I've been thinking that maybe medical school isn't right for me," she said after I questioned her about postcollege ambitions. "I know it's the thing I'm supposed to do, especially after having gone to Harvard, but I'm not sure."

"Really?" I asked. It was surprising, given that everyone else on the premed track talked incessantly about medical school.

"Yeah, what I really want is to help people," she answered, "to provide them with medical care. I have been looking into other career paths that would let me do that sooner rather than later, like becoming a physician assistant."

I had limited knowledge of the health-care field. "Is that like a doctor's helper or something?"

"No, not really like that," she explained with forgiving patience. "A physician assistant can basically do everything a doctor can do, but they have to be supervised by a doctor. They see patients, make diagnoses, and even write prescriptions in most states."

"Wow, that's cool. I've never heard of that."

"Yeah, and it's a two-year master's program," said Mia. "I'm just concerned about spending four years in med school, three years in residency, and then having to work for years to pay off all the debt."

"Wouldn't it bug you, though, not to have the authority of a doctor?"

"I guess it would depend on the doctor I worked with," she said. "Everything in life has a trade-off."

"I guess so," I agreed, although I hadn't thought much about trade-offs. My postcollege goal had been to find the highest-paying job.

Graduation came quickly. It was a heartbreaking good-bye, but we were headed in different directions. Mia was going home to New Jersey, having signed up for additional college classes at NYU. She had a few prerequisites to fulfill and would be applying to physician assistant programs in the fall.

We had agreed to keep in touch, but I was surprised when she phoned a week later. "Pat, I've been looking into things, and I could actually take these prereq classes at the University of Chicago in the fall."

"Really?" My heart skipped, my expectations for the future changing in an instant.

"Yeah, I'm pretty sure I could figure it out. But I wanted to talk about it first. We were pretty clear that we'd only date until graduation. I wanted to make sure you'd be okay with it."

"Okay with it?" I asked. "Are you kidding me? Yes, yes, definitely. Let's figure it out!"

"I've already done some looking. I'll have to fill out the application immediately . . ." Mia was providing details, but I was only half listening. I sensed a crucial turning point in my life.

Great new opportunities opened in front of me, and I couldn't have been happier.

***

When Mark and I arrived back in her room, Mia was sitting up in bed and nibbling vacantly at a turkey sandwich. She looked up but didn't register much emotion. They had given her an extra blanket, and she was wearing a navy sweatshirt I had brought along for her from Mark's house. Mia was usually cold, but the hospital itself was freezing.

"I see they finally found you some food?" asked Mark.

"Yes," she mumbled.

Just then Dr. Adams came into the room. "I'm on my way out, but I wanted to wait until you came back. Mark, we've completed all the tests. If you have a second, we can review things back in the office?"

"Sounds good," he said, turning to leave.

"Oh, Pat," said Dr. Adams, pausing before they left. "We gave Mia some more Ativan, quite a bit more than earlier. She should be feeling fairly comfortable now." She smiled, looking at Mia, and then they left.

I walked over to a chair next to the bed. Mia sat in silence, looking at her sandwich and taking a couple of small bites once in a while. I could tell that she was losing steam. I made a few comments, she murmured responses, and then we fell silent again. The beeping of machines was our only company.

After a half hour, Mark returned with a new doctor. He was solemn and tall with stern, intelligent eyes.

"Mia, Pat," introduced Mark, "this is a friend of mine, Dr. Patel."

I stood up to shake the doctor's hand. Mia glanced up but didn't say anything.

"Hello, Mia," began Dr. Patel in a deep voice. "I understand you haven't been sleeping much." He launched into the same questions that Mia had already answered several times that day. By this point, she was muttering short responses with an apathetic look. I jumped in with more complete answers, hoping that accurate details might help with a diagnosis.

After about fifteen minutes of this, Dr. Patel and Mark excused themselves, and our silent waiting continued. It was approaching 11:00 p.m., and the ER was deserted. This, combined with the low light, was making me sleepy, but it had little effect on Mia. She kept scanning the room, having given up on the half-eaten sandwich.

A nurse appeared, waking me from a stupor. "Hi, Mia," she said. "Dr. Patel prescribed a few more medications. I see you have some water there?"

She handed Mia a tiny paper cup containing three small pills. I had never seen Mia take medication without first knowing what it was. She downed them one by one without a second thought, a sign of her heavy sedation.

Given my conversation with Mark, I knew that at least one of those pills was for sleep. My own exhaustion was gone, and I became focused on watching Mia's eyes for any sign of drowsiness. She kept glancing around, looking at different areas of the ceiling.

Finally, after what seemed like an eternity, her eyes started to close. Suddenly, one of the machines made a noise, and she jolted awake. After a minute or two her eyelids started to droop again, but then another loud beep sounded.

This process continued for another twenty minutes, when I noticed the door slowly opening. Mark came half-way into the room and motioned for me to follow. Mia hadn't detected him. I stood up, gave her a light kiss on the forehead, and tiptoed into the hallway.

"Mark, she's almost asleep!" I whispered.

"Oh absolutely," he said, not bothering to lower his voice. "She won't be up much longer with all of that medi-cation. Come on, I want to go over some things while they move her. She's already been admitted."

He led me to a small office in the back of the ER. "Most everything came back normal," he said, sifting through papers. "Mia does have a bit of hypothyroidism. We can give her something for that, but I doubt it is causing the psychosis. She told us she took Relpax a few days ago. Do you know anything about that?"

"Yeah," I said, "that's her migraine medicine. She's been taking it for years."

"Right, and she's never had any reaction to it. So it can't be that, either."

"You're the doctor," I replied. "I just think she needs sleep."

"You could be right. Dr. Patel isn't sure, but he mentioned brief reactive psychosis. We'll have to see how she does tomorrow."

"What is that?" I asked. "'Brief reactive psychosis'?"

"People can become psychotic under periods of intense stress and anxiety," he answered. "It would be exacerbated by a lack of sleep. Their bodies can't handle the pressure."

"That's it!" I declared, smiling. "I'm sure that's it. How long does it last?"

"It can last up to thirty days, but Dr. Patel said that most cases resolve in twenty-four hours or a few days."

"Great, that's the best news I've heard in a long time."

"Let's hope so," said Mark. "In the interim, we have given her a small dose of an antipsychotic called Seroquel as well as another mood stabilizer, called Celexa. We'll also keep the Ativan going as needed, and we'll give her Restoril at night. That's the sleeping medication."

Mark led me to Mia's room on the hospital's third floor. She was already there, sound asleep in the darkness, finally looking peaceful. I had never been so happy to see someone sleeping.

He helped me unfold the visitor's chair into a make-shift bed, brought sheets and a blanket, and then told me that he would return in the morning. I thanked him again for everything and reached out for a handshake. Ignoring it, he gave me a quick hug and left.

Alone again, I plugged in my phone, which had run out of battery, and stood looking at Mia. She had a contented look on her face, and I was confident that her brain was repairing itself.

Turning back to my phone, I saw that my voice mail was filled with entries. The kids had left a message, saying how much they missed us. Mia's parents had left one a bit later, letting me know that the kids were asleep and everything was fine. My mom and Celia had also left messages.

The last one was from my brother, Brad, saying that he'd be up late. Even though it was past midnight, I tried him. He answered almost immediately. His wife, Jen, joined our conversation. They were two of our closest friends and knew Mia like a sister; the four of us had lived together right out of college. Brad and Jen wanted the full story, and I found it therapeutic to talk through the events of the day.

After the call, I stretched out on my temporary bed, relaxing in the comfort of Mia's rhythmic breathing. I wasn't tired yet, so I opened the phone's browser. I was curious about brief reactive psychosis and started researching it.

Everything I found supported Dr. Patel's diagnosis. The condition struck unexpectedly and in periods of intense stress, often in middle age. It affected more women than men, and many were the children of immigrants. I was halfway through reading the results of a scientific study when my eyelids finally started to close.

Mia will wake up as her old self, I promised myself, settling into a restless sleep. *We'll never have to deal with something like that again.*

The sounds of hospital machines continued to haunt me throughout the night, and the nurses returned regularly to take Mia's blood pressure. Fortunately, these distractions didn't bother her, but they kept waking me every hour or so. One time, when I was lying awake after one of these interruptions, she mumbled something in her sleep, but I couldn't make out what she was saying.

Mia woke shortly after 9:00 a.m. The nurses had gone, and I was the only one around when she opened her eyes. She sat up and looked around the room in confusion.

"Good morning," I said, standing to give her a kiss. "How are you feeling, babe?"

"I feel okay," she said, "a little tired." Her eyes had more life than the previous day, although she still seemed distant.

"That's not surprising," I replied. "Kind of a rough day yesterday."

"Yeah, I guess." Her tone was flat.

When Mark arrived, he greeted Mia and started to ask more piercing questions. Was she feeling tense and anxious? Did she think that the police were after her? She responded normally to everything, although she seemed more serious than usual.

I tried to lighten the mood by making a joke about how soundly she had slept, complaining that I had been tortured by machines all night. I also mentioned that she had talked in her sleep.

"What did I say?" asked Mia.

"I couldn't make it out," I said, "but it must have been a good dream. You seemed pretty worked up about something."

A nurse came in with more Ativan, which Mia begrudgingly swallowed. She complained of being groggy and feeling "out of it," and she didn't want to take more medication. But Mark implored her to continue, insisting that she had to follow Dr. Patel's orders.

I was in good spirits. Mia was acting as normal as possible under the circumstances. She was tired, and her personality was blunted given all the medication, but the psychotic ramblings were gone. Being around her wasn't the spooky, stressful experience that it had been the previous day.

Mia's parents brought the kids to the hospital shortly before lunch. I met them in the parking lot, and with open arms both Will and Jamie ran to me on the sidewalk. They were so excited, and I scooped them into a group hug.

"It's so great to see you two!" I gushed. "I've missed you so much!"

"Is Mommy all better now?" asked Jamie, not breaking our three-way embrace.

"Yes, and she's going to be so happy to see you both!"

As I stood up and the kids started walking toward the hospital, I greeted Marcos and Lucia. Mark had updated them on the details of Dr. Patel's diagnosis, and I could see the relief in their eyes, too.

On the way through the lobby, in the gift shop the kids picked up a teddy bear for Mia. The cheerful voices of a nine-year-old and eleven-year-old can certainly brighten an otherwise downcast hospital corridor. I felt like my world, the one that had been shattered the previous day, was piecing itself back together.

It didn't take long for Jamie to spot Mia. Fearless and determined, she ran straight through the room and right to Mia's side with her energetic greeting: "Mommy! Mommy!"

Will was more hesitant, slowing down to fully assess the hospital room with all of its technology and sounds. But once he saw Jamie hugging Mia, a huge grin lit up his face, and he ran over to join them.

I watched from across the room and noticed that Mia's excitement didn't match the moment. She hugged the kids, and she was talking to them, but she didn't show much enthusiasm. I chalked up the strange response to all the medication.

Marcos and Lucia greeted Mia in their restrained manner. Marcos asked a few questions about her medication, but Lucia seemed uncomfortable and timid. The kids wound up making plenty of noise for us all; they became fascinated by Mia's lunch tray, especially the red Jell-O and chocolate pudding.

After a short stay, Marcos and Lucia left to drive the kids back to our house in Sarasota, and then things quieted down again. Trying to lighten the mood, I said, "Well, we've been through better, and we've been through worse."

Mia turned to me, her face a grim reflection of its usual cheer. "Pat," she asked, "when have we ever been through worse?"

I smiled and grabbed her hand. "I guess you're right. But if we can get through that, we can get through anything."

She didn't acknowledge the comment. Instead, she asked, "What did I say last night, in my sleep?"

Something was strange in the way she asked it. "What?" I said, laughing it off. "I can't remember. You mentioned one of the doctors. You must have been dreaming about your work." I found her fixation on it odd, but just then Mark stopped in to suggest that Mia try to get some rest, so I let it go.

That afternoon, Mark, Dr. Patel, and I met in Mia's room for her psychiatric evaluation. Dr. Patel greeted her pleasantly and then started peppering her with questions. They started out routine. How did she feel? How had she slept? But then they turned more sinister. Did she feel paranoid? Did she feel like someone was out to get her? Did she hear any voices in her head? As she had done with Mark earlier, Mia answered as anyone would, without hesitation.

"Okay," said the physician after his questioning, "if what you are saying is true, Mia, I believe that you suffered from brief reactive psychosis. The stress from the changes at your work interrupted your sleeping patterns. The lack of sleep, combined with the additional pressure in your life, caused a chemical imbalance in your brain. I want you to take it easy for a while. Take at least a week away from work and get plenty of rest."

Mia was nodding as Dr. Patel spoke, her face unchanging, but a smile creased my lips. Hearing an expert confirm the diagnosis was a tremendous comfort.

"We have been giving you Ativan," he continued, "which as you know is an antianxiety medication. We also have you on a small dose of Seroquel, which is an antipsychotic drug. I'd like you to continue taking these medications until you have established a relationship with a psychiatrist in Sarasota. I'd also recommend taking

Restoril as needed at night. We need to make sure you get plenty of sleep."

Mia looked from the doctor to Mark and then over to me. I knew she didn't like being on so much medication, but I also knew that anything was better than suffering through another day like the previous one.

"Okay," she sighed.

"Good," said Dr. Patel. "I've asked them to keep you here one more night. I want to make sure we have your sleep back on track. If all goes well, you will be released tomorrow morning."

The nurse came in to take Mia's blood pressure, and Dr. Patel used it as his opportunity to say goodbye. As the nurse was distracting Mia, Mark grabbed my elbow and led me outside. Dr. Patel had stopped in the hallway, and he turned to face us.

"She seems much better, no disorganized thoughts or paranoia," said Mark.

"Yes, she does," agreed Dr. Patel. "Still, I'd like to be sure. Sometimes it can be hard to tell, as we can't see her thoughts for ourselves. Let's see how she does tonight. I won't be here in the morning, but the psychiatrist on duty can give her a final examination before she leaves."

Dr. Patel then turned to me. "It will be very important for your wife to see a psychiatrist when you get home. Someone needs to be monitoring her regularly and providing instruction on the medication."

The rest of the night was relaxed and uneventful. Mark went home while I stayed with Mia. Around 8:30 p.m., the nurse brought the little paper cup filled with pills.

"I hate being on all this medication," Mia said, looking down into the cup. "I don't feel right. My thinking feels dulled, and I'm so tired."

"Tired might be okay right now, babe," I said. "The doctor wanted you to get plenty of sleep."

"I guess so," she replied. She grabbed one of the pills. "This is the Seroquel. I never thought I'd be taking something like this."

I didn't know what to say. I opted for reassuring. "You heard the doctor; it was a onetime event. Yeah, it was bad, but it's over now, and our lives can go back to normal."

Mia looked from me back to the pill. She gulped it down and then grabbed the Restoril and Ativan. Less than an hour later, she was taking deep breaths and twitching. I put my ear to her mouth to hear her breathing, relishing the fact that she had fallen asleep so easily.

I woke early the next morning and drove back to Marcos and Lucia's house to pack our remaining things. Mia was still asleep when I left. When I returned a couple of hours later, she was up and talking with Mark. Apparently, I had just missed the attending psychiatrist, but Mark assured me that all had gone well and Mia would be released.

"Here," said Mark, handing me several forms. "These are her scripts. There is a pharmacy downstairs if you want to go fill them now." He walked me to the door.

"She seems good," he whispered when we reached the hallway, his face finally relaxing into a bright smile. "I'm pretty happy with the way this turned out."

"Me too." I returned his grin. "Thank God you were around for this, Mark. I honestly don't know what we would have done without you."

Within the hour, we had three bottles of new prescriptions and the all clear from the hospital. We said goodbye to Mark and started the drive home. Mia's mood hadn't changed from the previous night, but no one expected her to recover immediately.

That was a close one, I thought, studying the road ahead. I knew that accidents and tragedies are part of life. People would get sick; loved ones would die. But Mia and I were young, and the thought of losing her was unimaginable. I shuddered thinking about the brain tumor conversation. As hard as the weekend had been, it could have been much worse.

My wonderful wife was healthy again, and everything was going to be alright.

5

THE NIGHTMARE

Van Halen
"Ain't Talkin' 'Bout Love"
1:49–2:02

My cousin's wedding was held in my hometown shortly after Mia moved to Chicago. Dozens of aunts, uncles, and cousins would be attending. We had a big family, rowdy and loud.

Mia had no problem handling the weekend. A year later, when I met the extended Delgado clan in Miami, I would understand why. She had a lifetime of practice navigating hectic family reunions.

Outside of the crowded gatherings, we found time for more intimate conversations with members of my family. We spent one afternoon with my grandmother. Her mind was still sharp, as was her sense of humor, so visits with her were usually uplifting. But she had been widowed for years, and sometimes all she wanted was to reminisce about my grandfather and their many old friends, most of whom had died. I had always tried to change the subject when this happened. I was uncomfortable focusing on death and the passage of time.

Mia, never one to shy away from difficult topics, had a different approach. When the stories began, she leaned forward to listen. She sat close to my grandmother, holding her hand gently with sincere interest, asking questions and nodding patiently during the long answers. I was captivated watching their interaction.

As my focus shifted from Mia to my grandmother, a new understanding dawned. Although the stories made me sad, they meant everything to her. She cherished Mia's attention, savoring the fact that someone was giving her memories the respect they so properly deserved.

I will never forget the important lesson about compassion Mia taught me that afternoon. I realized that in her, I had found a person for whom kindness was as natural as taking a breath.

As we grew closer, it became clear that she and I both believed spending time with our loved ones was invaluable. And that set up another conversation I will never forget.

It was a Sunday morning sometime during our second winter in Chicago. I had been working long hours without a day off for three weeks. My brother, Brad, and his girlfriend at the time, Jen, shared an apartment with me. Mia had stayed over after meeting us in the city for a late dinner.

"Ugh," I groaned as the alarm sounded. "I can't believe that I have to go in to work right now." I was feeling down, jealous that they would be hanging out together all day. "You know, I would pay five thousand dollars if I could stay home with you three today."

"Wow, Pat, you need to get your priorities straight," Mia answered. "Why don't you calculate what you are actually making per hour. I bet five thousand dollars is over a month's worth of your time."

I stopped, having never thought about it that way, but she was right. I was willing to forfeit more than a month's worth of wages to buy back a single day for myself. I cannot emphasize enough the impact that her comment had on me. It started me down the long but important path of self-discovery. How should I spend my time? What was most important to me?

Finding answers to these questions would take years, but one thing was certain. Whatever I did, and wherever I ended up, I wanted Mia to be with me.

***

When we pulled into the garage at the end of our drive home, I immediately noticed the sign taped to the door. "Welcome Home!" it read, with a cute drawing of a house and the sun shining above it. Will and Jamie had been busy preparing our arrival.

They came running with cheers when we walked in. "You're home!" they cried, our little dog barking loudly in their wake.

Mia had walked in first, but she didn't say much. She bent to hug them, muttered a despondent greeting, and wandered off. Instead, they shifted their focus to me. "Yes, we are home!" I whooped, kneeling down to their level and sharing their enthusiasm. Soon, all three of us were chasing the dog excitedly around the house.

After my romp with the kids, I reconnected with Mia. My in-laws were preparing dinner, which gave us time to handle a few important tasks.

In our study, with the door closed, we held a video call with Mia's cousin Alex, the psychiatrist from Miami. He was Mark's age, with short-cropped hair and tan skin. He was confident and earnest, his speech accented by the Spanish intonations so prevalent in the English spoken throughout Miami.

Our conversation lasted about thirty minutes. At one point, Alex asked Mia if she could remember anything from Sunday. "I remember some of it," she said. "What I remember most is that my mind was racing nonstop."

"Yeah," said Alex, "that does happen. I've heard people refer to it as a 'tornado of ideas' swirling inside their head."

"That's exactly how it felt, like I had an unstoppable tornado spinning in my brain, and I couldn't do anything about it."

It was hard to imagine how scary it must have been for Mia to lose control of her thoughts like that.

Alex also asked about her treatment plan. "Rest and medication," she moaned. "I don't like taking the pills. I don't feel like myself."

"No one likes it, but you have to keep taking them," Alex responded. "It's the most powerful tool that we have."

"I know it's important," she groused.

"What do they have you on?"

"Ativan, Restoril, and Seroquel, but honestly, I'm not sure of the doses." She looked at me.

I had a small notebook that I was using to track our instructions. I opened it and read off the information that I had scribbled. "Mia is taking two milligrams of

Ativan three to four times a day, twenty-five milligrams of Seroquel twice a day, and then fifteen to thirty milligrams of Restoril before bed for sleep."

"Wow, really?" Alex asked. "Mia, you must weigh about a hundred pounds. I can't believe you're not sleeping now. The Seroquel dose seems low, but even so that regimen should keep you pretty tired."

"Well, that's what Dr. Patel wanted," I said, "to keep her tired."

"That makes sense," said Alex, "and given that Mia is so thin, the extra pounds shouldn't be an issue." I caught this last comment but didn't think much of it. I had no experience with these kinds of pharmaceuticals, and I wasn't aware that most of them caused significant weight gain.

He then started commenting on other drugs, many with names I had never heard. I tried to keep track of them all—Abilify, Risperdal, Lexapro—before it became too much. But he wasn't recommending them; it was more like he was discussing various alternatives with himself. Before hanging up, he agreed to help us find a good psychiatrist in Sarasota.

Next, we had to address Mia's work situation. The acquisition of her physician group would be consummated in two days, and she had to decide if she would be accepting a position in the new company. Her response was already overdue.

As we discussed it, I could tell that Mia was hesitant. She loved her work, but she was scared. She didn't want to risk a return to the emergency room. I didn't want that, either. And I didn't want her stewing over the decision when she should be resting.

"Look, babe," I said, "given everything that has happened, what about taking a break for a while?"

Relief eased the tension in her face as she nodded. I helped her draft a reply, one that would leave the door open for future employment but would turn down the immediate opportunity. When I say that I helped, what I mean is that I wrote the email, and she sat beside me, watching.

I carefully crafted an excuse that was neither dishonest nor forthright. It certainly didn't include any mention of the explicit issue. Regretfully, my reaction was all too common when it came to mental illness: I hid the truth. I was hoping to shield Mia from the accompanying stigma.

Looking back, I should have contacted one of the doctors in her practice and had a heart-to-heart conversation, but in the moment, and without experience, I did what I thought was best for Mia and her career. I had just witnessed Mark, who was also a medical professional, go to incredible lengths to keep her out of a mental health facility.

We were lucky to keep things secret, I told myself. *No one but our closest family members can ever know what really happened.*

That night I lay patiently beside Mia, willing her to fall asleep. When she finally began twitching, I snuck out of the bedroom. So many people had left voice mails, from all sides of our family, that I felt compelled to provide updates. It was well past midnight when I finally climbed back into bed, thoroughly exhausted.

Wednesday started as a typical day. I spent the morning at the office, catching up on work I had been neglecting. Late in the afternoon, I met Mia at an appointment with an ear specialist for Jamie.

Walking into the waiting room, I found Mia and her mom sitting quietly with Jamie. Lucia was acting as a temporary chauffeur, given that Mia wasn't supposed to be driving while so heavily medicated. I greeted them and sat down.

After a couple of minutes, the receptionist asked Mia to come up to the desk. Mia gave me a strange glance like, *Why does she need to see me?* I shrugged and kind of nodded my head like, *I don't know, why don't you go find out?*

She continued to look puzzled as she made her way to the window, and I suddenly felt uneasy. It wasn't like her. She worked in a doctor's office; she knew the way things worked.

She returned with a clipboard and several forms. She sat staring at them, a grimace across her face.

"What's the matter, babe?" I whispered nervously. "You look troubled."

"This is ridiculous, why does *she* need this information?" Mia demanded in a low tone.

I glanced at the paperwork, which appeared standard. It requested the typical information, like name, date of birth, and type of insurance. Trying to sound casual, I said, "Looks like the regular stuff. You know, all doctors' offices ask for this sort of thing."

"Yes, but why does *she* need it?" repeated Mia, glaring at the receptionist, who was busy talking on the phone.

"Well, she doesn't personally," I said. "She wants us to fill it out for the doctor."

"No, she said, '*I* need you to fill this out for *me*.' That's what she said."

"Okay, well, that's not what she meant. She meant that she needs the information because it's part of their office protocol." I kept my voice calm and discreet, hoping that other people weren't following our conversation.

"Well, I'm not going to do it," snapped Mia, shoving the forms at me. "Here, you do it."

Obviously, something was wrong. I wondered if it could be the medication—changing her personality as it fought to stabilize the chemical balance in her brain. Or could she be suffering from the early phases of psychosis again, where she couldn't accurately interpret language? The thought sent a chill through me.

I filled out the forms, turned them in, and a half hour later we were seeing the doctor. Typically, Mia would have asked a number of incisive questions associated with Jamie's health, all of them grounded in an impressive repository of pediatric knowledge. Instead, she remained silent while I stumbled my way through the meeting.

After returning home, I pulled my mother-in-law aside. "Lucia, have you noticed anything strange about Mia's behavior today?"

"No, Pat," she said, her Cuban accent making it sound more like *Paht*. "Mia has been tired, and maybe a little impatient, but not like what we experienced at Celia's house." Her response gave me a little comfort, but not much.

In bed that night, I realized that a pattern was emerging. Mia would fall asleep almost exactly forty-five minutes after taking the Restoril. Once she did, I snuck out of the room again, this time to update Mark.

Through several texts, I informed him of the strange exchange at the doctor's office. He didn't like the sound of it but was pleased to hear that she was sleeping.

The next morning at work, I received a text from Mia. She was taking her mom for a tour of our church's youth program, and she wanted me to join them. It seemed a bit strange at the time but not entirely out of place. Mia had been active in youth education at the church for years. She had recently started teaching in the program for older kids and was excited about her new role.

I phoned Mark on my way to meet them. He wanted to know if I had arranged an appointment with a local psychiatrist.

"Yes, I called yesterday. Alex gave me the name of Dr. Johnny Martinez. We have an appointment with him on Monday."

"Dude, what? That's in four days!"

"Yeah, well, that's the earliest they could get us in. I told them it was important."

"It's not important," he cried, "it's urgent! Pat, you remember what Dr. Patel said. For all we know, Mia could be acting normal but thinking crazy shit. She needs to be under the care of someone with expert training. Now! She just got out of the emergency room!"

He caught me off guard. Did he think that I wasn't taking the situation seriously?

"Mark, what do you want me to do, demand that Martinez see us today?"

"Absolutely, a hundred percent that's what I want! Look, buddy, you're doing a great job. But I'm not a psychiatrist, and neither are you. We're guessing. Just get her in to see someone there immediately, okay? Do whatever you have to do."

"Okay, yeah, of course I will," I answered as I pulled into the church's parking lot. Mark was nervous, and it made me apprehensive. I resolved to contact Dr. Martinez's office as soon as possible.

The youth program was held in a small one-story building across the street from the sanctuary. I walked the halls lined with classrooms and found Mia and her mom in one of the far rooms. The walls were decorated with cartoons and Bible verses, and Mia was pointing to something at the back of the class. I greeted them both and then listened while Mia continued talking about a recent lesson. A few moments later, an older woman appeared at the door.

"Hi there, I just wanted to see who was here in our room," she said.

"What? No, this is *my* room," declared Mia. "*I* teach in this room." She said it aggressively, like she was defending her honor. My pulse quickened.

"Oh, I see," said the woman. "That's fine. Of course, we use this room for other things, too, you know?"

"Oh really?" snapped Mia. "And who are you?" She glanced over and gave me a disgusted look like, *Can you believe the gall of this lady?*

"I'm one of the new sisters here," the woman replied kindly. "I'm not sure we have met."

"Yes, hi, it's nice to meet you," I interjected, striding over quickly with an outstretched hand. "I'm Pat Dylan, and this is my wife, Mia, and my mother-in-law, Lucia. Mia teaches here in the catechism program. She was just showing us around."

"Ah, and we thank you for that, dear," said the nun, smiling at Mia while shaking my hand. "I'm Sister Mary. I'm pleased to be part of the parish. I moved here last month."

The wife I knew would have beaten me to the greeting, probably given the sister a hug, and then chatted with her for a half hour. Instead, Mia stood on the far side of the room, scowling our way.

At this point, my heart was racing. I had to get Mia back to our house as quickly as possible.

"Right, well, please give our regards to Father John, whom we know well," I said, dropping the name of the senior priest and hoping it would defuse the situation. Thankfully, it worked. The woman made a few more comments and then left.

Mia remained upset, and I asked her to ride home with me. I wanted to keep her close and evaluate how she was thinking.

"Can you believe the nerve of that woman?" she snarled when we were alone in the car.

"Mia, that was just a nun checking to see who was walking around the building on a Thursday morning." I tried to sound nonchalant. My breathing had become rushed, and I was struggling to slow it down.

"No, she was saying that the room wasn't mine, Pat." Mia's eyes narrowed and her chin jutted forward. "That's *my* room. I teach in there. I taught there last week."

"I know," I pleaded, "but how would she know that? You just started teaching, and she's new to the parish."

Mia didn't respond. She was staring at me, wondering if I was on her side. I decided to end the discussion, trying hard to ignore the knot building in my stomach.

When we arrived home, Lucia was already in the kitchen. She must have noticed the strange behavior at the church, and she quickly offered to prepare lunch. I hastily led Mia into our room.

I closed the door and inhaled deeply, attempting to calm myself. Sitting her down on the bed, I said, "Babe, I'm worried about you. How are you feeling?"

"What do you mean? I feel fine. I'm just mad at that woman from the church. Who was she, and what was she trying to do?"

"We've been over this. She's a new nun in the parish, that's all."

"That's what she says, but who is she really?" Her eyes narrowed again. "What is God trying to tell us?"

The gates restraining my worst nightmare finally collapsed, despair flooding over me. It shouldn't be happening—*it couldn't be happening!* The delusions were back, even with Mia taking all the medication!

I forgot about everything but the next moment: keep Mia in our room, safe and protected. I could worry about the rest after that.

"Okay, well, maybe it's best if we try to relax," I replied, ignoring her question. "How about I change out of these work clothes, and we try to take a nap?"

"If you want to." Her expression made it clear that she found the request a strange one.

I quickly changed into shorts and a T-shirt. We had a CD player in our room and a pile of discs strewn about. I grabbed a Van Morrison album and put it on. I turned off the lights and lay down with my head on the pillow. Mia followed my lead.

Lying there, I wondered if she could hear my heart pounding. I knew she wasn't going to fall asleep, but I needed time to think. Mark was no longer around, and a trip to the emergency room was not an option. My pulse thumped against my eardrums as the first song ended.

"Pat, what did I say in my sleep that night in the hospital?" Mia asked suddenly. She was staring, wide eyed, up at the ceiling.

"I can't remember. Why?"

"I think it might be important," she said, without looking at me.

"It wasn't important. You were talking in your sleep."

"I think it has to do with the numbers 3, 6, 8, and 9, but I can't work it out." She said it matter-of-factly, without any hint of humor.

"Okay, well, try to work that out," I said softly. "I'll be back in a second." I grabbed my phone, hands shaking, and walked into the hall. Closing the door, I shut my eyes and leaned against the wall, slowly exhaling several deep breaths.

Mia needs you, I kept repeating to myself. *Keep it together.*

"Marcos, Lucia," I said as I entered the kitchen, "Mia isn't doing well. We're going to be in our bedroom for a while. Can you call Mark and tell him that things are worse than I thought? I'll update him when I can."

I needed time to contact Dr. Martinez's office and convince him to see Mia immediately, but I was worried about leaving her alone too long. I decided to give her more Ativan. Maybe that would help her relax, or at least keep her sedated. I didn't know what else to do.

When I returned to our bedroom, Van Morrison was singing his song "*Sweet Thing.*" It had always been one of our favorites. Mia was propped up on her pillow, waiting for me.

"When he wrote this song, he was thinking of us," she said. "I'm sure of it."

"Mia, we have never met Van Morrison. He couldn't have been thinking of us."

"No," she said in a firm voice, "I am telling you that he was thinking of us."

"He wrote this song in 1968, babe," I replied. "Neither one of us was born then."

I stood watching her from across the room. Mia rose slowly and marched over. She stopped about a foot away, glaring up at me. I had the fleeting feeling that she was going to punch me. "You need to tell me what I said the other night, in my sleep, at the hospital."

I was not seeing my best friend across from me. I couldn't recognize her, like she was someone else.

"Why." It wasn't a question. I stated it, daring her to respond.

"It was important. I know it," she said in the same grave tone.

A heartbeat. And then another.

"Mia, do you think that whatever you said that night was a message from God, and that it will solve the meaning of those numbers that you just mentioned?" I couldn't believe I was actually saying this.

Her stare was boring into me. There was no sign of Mia in those eyes; they were void of intimacy. For a brief second, just a flash, I might have seen a flicker of hesitation, or maybe it was remorse, but then it was gone.

"Yes," she said. "That's exactly what I think."

6.

THE TRUTH

Poi Dog Pondering
"Catacombs"
2:37–3:15

My illness struck when Mia and I first began living in Chicago. I developed a dull pain in my abdomen. It felt as if someone were perpetually twisting a blunt knife into my stomach.

Back then, I believed that physicians had all the answers. If you got sick, you had only to find the right doctor. He or she would give you the appropriate pill or surgery, and you would be fine. But this new disease was different. I saw many doctors, and no one had any answers. Tests came back negative; scans and MRIs turned up nothing.

I was in constant pain. Physically, it was difficult; mentally, it was devastating. When you are trapped in a body that refuses to heal, your mind doesn't know how to cope. All you want is to be healthy again, but nothing you do brings you any closer to that goal.

A year into my ordeal, a doctor suggested that I try taking a steroid called prednisone. He didn't know what was ailing me, but the drug was used to treat inflammation across a range of afflictions. He thought it might help. He was reaching, but I was desperate.

After being on prednisone for a week, my condition deteriorated rapidly. Combined with my already weakened immune system, it triggered a bizarre infection of my mouth and throat. I became delirious, with a dangerously high fever. The steroid was exacerbating my illness, but I couldn't stop taking it. It was so powerful that the dose could only be slowly decreased over time.

Mia came to my rescue. She dropped everything to remain by my side, kneeling by the bed as I suffered in a half-comatose state. I would slide in and out of delirium, waking to find her placing a cool cloth on my forehead or simply holding my hand and watching over me.

At one point, the situation became so unstable that she rushed me to the hospital. I have memories of huddling in the emergency room and hearing her take charge of my care.

"His fever spiked this morning, and he's thoroughly dehydrated." She was lecturing one of the medical assistants, responding with authority to his comments. "No, a glass of water won't help. His throat is so swollen that he can't swallow. He needs IV fluids, and he needs them *stat!*"

Once the steroid was tapered down, the infection cleared. The whole ordeal took another week, a week in which Mia did nothing but concentrate on my health.

When it was over, she was adamant. "We aren't treating symptoms anymore, Pat," she said. "We need to identify the cause of this."

"Isn't that what doctors are for?" I asked.

"Maybe," she replied, "but it's your health." She decided that together we could find a cure for my illness, even if no one else believed it possible.

Mia never once faltered in her belief that we would find a way to treat my condition.

***

My wife was psychotic again, and for a moment I froze, helpless against the mysterious illness.

I needed a plan of attack. First, I had to get Mia to a psychiatrist. What we were doing was definitely not working. Second, I had to keep her as isolated as possible. I didn't want the kids to see her like this; it would be too disturbing. Plus, given the stigma of mental illness, I wanted to protect her from rumors that might spread if word of her condition leaked out. Finally, in the short term, I had to sedate her so that she didn't become too aggressive or loud, as had happened in Celia's garage.

But at the moment, Mia was standing in front of me, a defiant expression on her face.

"Mia, I have told you this already," I pleaded. "I don't remember exactly what you said in your sleep that night. It sounded like you were replying to a comment that one of the doctors made. You said something like, 'I wrote it in the file.'"

That seemed to satisfy her. She walked back over and sat on the bed. She put a finger to her mouth and copped an inquisitive look, like she was trying to solve yet another riddle. "I wrote it in the file . . . in the file . . . single file . . . numbers in single file . . ."

She kept talking, but I wasn't listening. I was trying to find the Ativan. Dr. Patel had said to give it as needed, and it was definitely needed now.

Somehow, I convinced Mia to take the medication and lie down again. She complied, but she kept going on about the numbers and the message from God. "Pat, I need to know exactly what happened and when. We need to go over everything from the start."

"Okay, right," I agreed. "That's a good idea. Why don't you get going on that, and I'll be back in a few minutes? I'm going to call work and let them know I won't be in this afternoon."

I returned to the kitchen; Marcos and Lucia were still sitting at the table. "Mia is suffering from psychosis again. It's the same as it was Sunday." I said it matter-of-factly, and I think they expected it. Lucia must have told Marcos about the incident at church. "I'm going to keep her in our room as much as possible. Can you handle the kids after school and dinner and all that?"

"Yes, Pat," replied Marcos. "We will do anything you need us to do." Mia's parents looked concerned and scared, but they trusted me.

I walked to the back of the house, where we had a big family room. It was packed with toys, musical instruments, couches, and a television. It was also the farthest room from our bedroom, and I didn't want Mia to overhear my conversation when I called Dr. Martinez's office.

"My wife has gotten a lot worse since yesterday," I explained when the receptionist answered. "She's completely psychotic again."

"I'm so sorry to hear that, Mr. Dylan," she responded. "If this is an emergency, you should hang up and dial 911."

"No, it's not an emergency like that," I said, trying to sound like I knew what I was talking about, "but it is urgent. I really need Dr. Martinez to see her as soon as possible. Is there any chance that I can bring her in this afternoon?"

"I'm sorry, sir," she said, "but Dr. Martinez is not in the office this afternoon."

I remembered the conversation with Mark and had the brief thought of demanding to see the doctor immediately, but then I quickly dismissed it. My only hope was to appeal to this woman's sympathy.

"Oh, that's too bad. How about tomorrow?" I asked. "Can you somehow fit us in tomorrow?" I was being as polite as possible, but desperation filled my voice. "My wife is really struggling. I can't tell you how much it would mean to me."

The long silence meant the receptionist was trying to find a solution. "Um, okay, let's see," she eventually said. "Why don't you come in at 1:00 p.m. tomorrow? I'll talk to Dr. Martinez and see if he can make that work."

"Oh, thank you. Thank you so much." I only had to manage Mia through the next twenty-four hours, and that seemed doable. Unfortunately, my confidence lasted until I opened the door to our bedroom. Mia was on the phone and appeared frustrated.

"What do you mean?" she thundered. "Why don't you just answer my question!"

I couldn't believe that I had forgotten to take her cell phone. Here I wanted to isolate her, and I left her sitting within easy reach of the entire world.

Mia noticed that I had returned. "I have to go!" she barked, putting down the phone.

"Who was that?" I asked casually.

"No one," she retorted, frowning at me. "I want to talk to you, Pat. I want *the truth*." She looked furious.

"The truth about what, babe?" I tried to act relaxed even though my palms were sweating.

"I want you to tell me the truth about *everything*." Her response was slow, her voice loud and firm.

"Mia, I wish I had the answers to everything, I really do. But I don't." I said it with a forced smile, pretending like we both knew that what she was requesting was impossible. "Before I left, you wanted to review what had happened, didn't you?"

"Yes, I did," she replied, her demeanor suddenly changing. My muscles relaxed slightly. Maybe I could manage her like a toddler, changing the subject when necessary.

"Okay, let's grab a piece of paper, and we can go through things," I suggested. She seemed interested in this new line of discussion, so I wasted no time in snatching my notebook and pencil.

We spent the next hour reviewing the events of the past week in excruciating detail. We had to list incidents chronologically, broken down into fifteen-minute segments. Mia had always been meticulous, and she approached this like a scientist recording the results of an experiment:

> Sunday, 5:30 a.m.: wake up Pat, concerned about prison
>
> Sunday, 5:45 a.m.: get into shower

Sunday, 6:00 a.m.: start getting ready for church

Many times, she would demand that we go back to the beginning to make sure we hadn't missed anything. She didn't remember much from Sunday or Monday, but she was certain that clues were hidden in the past, so she kept asking the same questions over and over. It took every ounce of my patience.

After an hour, it appeared that the Ativan was kicking in. She no longer seemed as angry, but her thoughts were becoming more scattered. She kept hopping around the conversation like,

"What happened after we arrived at the emergency room?"

"Well, then you went back with Mark while I filled out the paperwor—"

"What kind of bird is that out back?"

"It looks like a—"

"Is that a stain on the drapes over there, or is that blood?"

"It can't be blood, it must be—"

"Why can't it be blood, Pat? What do *you* know about those drapes?"

After this last accusation, I rubbed my eyes with my hands in frustration.

"Why did you do that, with your hands right there? Why did you do that?"

That was our afternoon, going around and around in circles. At times, she would become hung up on specific words, finding links among them that weren't there. It was like playing connect the dots with homonyms. She would say things like, "Look at that pair of shoes. I need to pare down my thoughts. I think I have a pear in the kitchen. No, someone ate it. Eight. 3, 6, 8, and 9. Those are the numbers: 3, 6, 8, and 9 . . ."

At one point, I proposed watching a movie, hoping it might help to focus her attention. We had a television in our room, and I noticed a disc lying nearby. She half-heartedly agreed, so I put in the film. It was the animated movie *Up*.

I had never seen *Up* and had no idea what it was about. In the first ten minutes, a couple grows old together and then the wife dies. That started Mia talking about death, about how one of us was going to die before the other. She was trying to figure out which one of us would go first, like maybe those special numbers had something to do with it. "Will I die first? 3, 6, 8, and 9. Nine. Nine. Is that right? *Nein*. I don't know whether it is. Check the weather. It looks like rain. Someone needs to take the reins . . ."

Quickly turning it off, I suggested instead that we watch home videos. We had taken hours of movies of the kids when they were little, and we had them all nicely organized by the bed. I hoped they would keep thoughts of death and secret connections out of her head.

As the movie started, a three-year-old Will ran around the house in a Spider-Man costume. A one-year-old Jamie followed closely behind, dressed like a fairy princess with wings and a magic wand. Our little dog raced after them both, barking loudly.

"Look at Celia, she's so frustrated that Luke is getting all the attention," sighed Mia, not realizing that she had replaced our kids' names with those of her two youngest siblings. I let it go; correcting her didn't seem necessary. But as the movie played on, she became even more confused.

"I should have given Celia more attention," she said. "I really should have. Wait, is that Luke? No, that looks like Will." She stared at the screen intently, concentration creasing her face. "It must be Luke. No, no . . . that looks like Will."

"Yeah, that's Will and Jamie, babe. These are our home movies, not your parents'."

She was upset that she had made the mistake and wanted the movie turned off. It was too difficult for her to follow. We reverted to poring over events of the prior week. I kept glancing at the clock, like a student in class who can't wait for the bell to ring. We heard the kids return from school, but we never left the room.

After a while, I sensed that Mia was aware that something was wrong. I used the opportunity to broach the use of her phone, suggesting that she limit calls to only her closest friends. She agreed, and we wrote down the people she could contact. It wasn't a long list, and I hoped it would curtail her external communications.

When Lucia finally knocked on the door to tell us that dinner was ready, I was willing to chance an interaction with the kids. My mind was exhausted from trying to follow the thoughts racing through Mia's troubled mind, and I needed the escape.

I greeted Will and Jamie in the kitchen, but Mia remained subdued, barely addressing them. The food was already on the table, so we all sat down. I was watching Mia closely; it was taking all of her willpower to stay quiet.

Jamie's imagination usually came alive at the dinner table. She was talkative and liked to share whatever had transpired at school that day. "Let's play high-low," she suggested. High-low was a game we played most nights. It consisted of going around the table with everyone saying both the best and the worst thing that had happened to them that day. "I'll start!"

"Okay," I said, hoping that Jamie's talent for make-believe wouldn't become an issue.

"My high was: I found out I have a superpower today!" She smiled broadly. "I can hover off the ground. Watch this. Just watch my feet, and you'll see!" She stood up, putting a hand on the chair to either side of her. She then used her arms to push herself up, bringing her feet off the ground. "See? See my feet? I'm flying!"

Usually, Mia and I would play along, exclaiming that we always knew that she was a superhero and bragging about what lucky parents we were. Instead, my reaction was muted, and Mia was scandalized. She was looking from Jamie to me and then back to Jamie again.

"Oh, Celia, you don't really have the ability to fly," she said. She turned to me. "Pat, she doesn't really think she can fly, does she?"

"No, she doesn't think that," I muttered, feeling awful. Jamie was devastated and certainly noticed that Mia had used the wrong name. "But you know our *Jamie*, she definitely has superpowers!" I said, tousling Jamie's hair and stressing her name.

The game stalled after the kids realized that their mom was acting weird. We finished the rest of the meal in a combination of broken conversation and awkward silence.

After dinner, Mia and her mom returned to our room. Lucia had offered to take over so that I could spend time with the kids.

I always read to them before bed. That night, after they were ready and settled, I paused before launching into the book. "Have either of you noticed that Mom hasn't really been acting like herself?" I asked, unsure if I was making a parenting mistake. But I knew that in their position, I would want answers.

I looked first to Will. He sat silently, but I saw relief on his face. He was clearly thankful that I had broached the subject. Jamie was fidgeting with her sheets, perhaps still feeling the sting from the game of high-low.

"I only ask because . . . well, I have noticed," I admitted. "That's why I was home today with her while you were at school."

"Mom was already in the hospital," Will whispered. "I thought she was all better."

"Yeah, that's what Uncle Mark and I thought, too." I tried to sound as confident and soothing as possible. "But sometimes, you know, when we get sick, we might think we're better, but we still have some of the sickness lingering around."

"Sometimes I have a runny nose even after my sore throat goes away," said Jamie, helpfully trying to support my argument.

"Right, and that's what Mom has right now. Well, not really a *runny nose*," I said, attempting to get a laugh by implying that runny noses were gross. They both giggled a little.

"Look," I said, "you know how when you have a cold, and your nose isn't working right—it's either runny or it's stuffed up, and you can't control it?" They were both nodding. "Well, that's what's going on with Mom right now.

It's like she has a cold, but the cold isn't in her nose, it's in her brain."

"She has a cold in her brain?" asked Jamie, trying desperately to follow my explanation.

"Well, not actually a cold, but like a cold," I replied. "What it means is that Mom's brain isn't working properly right now, and she can't control it. She's still the same Mom who loves you more than anything, though. She just isn't acting like herself right now."

"Okay," said Jamie, who seemed satisfied with the explanation. Will sat looking down at the pillow he was sitting on.

"But she's going to get better, I promise, just like you get better every time you have a cold," I vowed. "It's going to take some time, though, and so we have to be patient with her. You know how she's always patient with you when you're sick?"

They were both nodding again. "So, let's be as patient as we can and remember that Mom really needs our help right now." I was going to leave it at that, but then I added, "Oh, and one more thing, let's keep Mom's sickness to ourselves. It will be our secret, okay?"

Looking back, this last part was shameful. I was reinforcing the stigma, teaching our kids that mental illness shouldn't be discussed openly.

"Right. Now, it's time for a group hug and then on with the story!" I exclaimed in a happy voice, oblivious to the inexcusable way that I had ended the conversation.

Later that night, after the Restoril had taken effect, I crept to the back room and started dialing every person on Mia's contact list. It included her closest friends, not only from Sarasota but also from college and her hometown in New Jersey.

A half dozen people were on the list. For some, I left a message and followed up with an email. A few answered my call, and I provided a full update. I tried to keep the conversations short, given that it was past 10:00 p.m., but it wasn't easy. Understandably, Mia's friends were in shock. It felt good, enlisting other trusted individuals in my crusade to support her.

By the time I crawled back into bed beside Mia, it was past 1:00 a.m. It was my first chance to relax all day. Lying there in the silence of our room, I relished the tranquility. I knew it wouldn't last.

The next morning, after seeing the kids off to school, the torture with Mia began again. She continued to believe that clues to some kind of cosmic puzzle were hidden in the past. Mia was now scrutinizing an actual calendar day by day, recording every detail. This included not only the events of the recent week but also several weeks prior.

Her thoughts remained scattered, and she jumped from one idea to the next. We talked about memories from her childhood, things that had happened at Harvard, and incidents with the kids. We would kind of hover over an issue for a while, and then we'd abruptly skip to another topic. Periodically, she would stop and brusquely demand *the truth.*

Once, when I was a kid, my parents took us to Mexico. As the taxi pulled into our beachside resort, I saw a row of security guards holding machine guns. I didn't feel immediately threatened; the guns weren't pointed at me. But the atmosphere had a sense of potential combustion, like one wrong move and the bullets would start flying. It was the same sensation being trapped in a room with my psychotic wife.

By the time we were in the car headed to Dr. Martinez's office, I had become more experienced in dealing with the situation. I kept my movements to an absolute minimum. Any action of my limbs or turning of my head would trigger Mia. She would try to find the underlying meaning in anything and everything. If the tenor of my voice changed, or even if I sighed, it would instigate an investigation:

"You just scratched your cheek, why did you do that?"

"Um, because I had an itch there."

"Why the hesitation, Pat? Why won't you tell me *the truth?*"

It was an acquired skill, concentrating mightily to stay absolutely still, talk without emotion, and carefully choose every single word. The guise took effort, but it was certainly easier than dealing with the repercussions.

Walking into Dr. Martinez's lobby was my first experience with a psychiatrist's office. I have found that they are all similar. You have the quiet receptionist to greet you and wave you into the waiting area. This usually consists of a leather couch, a couple of chairs, and a table. On the wall, you will see comforting pictures of landscapes or sunsets with phrases like "Take the time to smile" or "Tomorrow is another day." And then there is the noise machine; there's always the noise machine. The sounds of white noise or falling water cover any voices that might leak out of the doctor's office. They also give the patient something to concentrate on instead of searching for the underlying meaning in every sound.

After ten minutes, Dr. Johnny Martinez came into the waiting room and greeted us. He was about our age, in his late thirties or early forties, thin and athletic looking. He seemed jovial, guiding us with a smile into his office. Mia and I sat together on a couch facing his desk.

"So, how are you feeling today, Mia?" he asked.

Mia's response was haphazard. He asked a couple of other questions. She was meandering through disjointed thoughts, telling him about her search for hidden meanings. I sat quietly, without moving a muscle. He must have noticed my discomfort; he kept glancing at me while Mia struggled through her answers.

Finally, Dr. Martinez turned my way. Mia was in midsentence, but he kind of cut her off. He picked up a whiteboard.

"Pat, this is what is happening. I want to explain it to you." He grabbed a black marker, drawing a person's head and then outlining a brain inside. "Let's say this is your wife's brain."

Mia looked angry. She didn't like being ignored and was trying to get his attention.

I gave him a wondering look like, *Why aren't you talking to Mia, too?* He dismissed my glance with a shake of his head. "She's not going to remember any of this, so I am telling it to you. You are the one who needs to hear it."

"Okay," I said, hoping that Mia didn't see it as some sort of betrayal.

"As I was saying, let's say this is your wife's brain. The way the brain functions is through neurotransmitters. There are a whole lot of these, but I want to focus on just two, dopamine and serotonin."

He grabbed a green marker and started writing little *D*'s across his cartoon brain. He then switched to a red marker and added little *S*'s. "This is a normal-functioning brain. You see how the dopamine and serotonin balance each other out?"

"Yes." I liked the way he was explaining it, simple but not patronizing.

"Well, in your wife's case, that is not happening." He started to erase the *S*'s until only a few were left. He then grabbed the green marker and added a bunch more *D*'s. "Your wife's brain has an overabundance of dopamine, and it's causing her thought disorder and paranoia."

"Okay, so what do we do?" Mia had given up trying to get Dr. Martinez's attention, but she wasn't listening to his explanation. She seemed focused on the light fixtures.

"How much Seroquel did you say she was taking?"

"She's taking twenty-five milligrams twice a day."

"No, that's not nearly enough. I want her taking six hundred milligrams per day."

"What?" I cried. "Dr. Martinez, that is more than ten times her current dose!"

"I am aware of that," he said. "Has your wife struggled with depression?"

"No, she hasn't. I mean, she felt down for a week or two after our son was born, but nothing major."

"That doesn't really count," he said, pulling a huge book off the shelf. It was the first time I had seen that particular book, but it wouldn't be the last. It was called the *Diagnostic and Statistical Manual of Mental Disorders*, or *DSM* for short. It was the holy grail of answers for mental health practitioners. It included descriptions for every accepted mental illness. "Interesting," he commented.

"What's interesting?" I liked Dr. Martinez and wanted to learn more from him.

"I'd be willing to bet that your wife has bipolar disorder. I mean, this looks like classic manic psychosis." He was talking to me while flipping through the large textbook. "There it is. Yep, that's what I thought." He glanced up with a look of concentration. "One doesn't need to suffer from mania to be bipolar. You need only have depression to be considered bipolar. But mania alone doesn't do it."

"Okay . . . but I'm not following."

"Your wife is manic. At least, that's how she is presenting. But she doesn't suffer from depression. The *DSM* would say, therefore, that she is not bipolar."

"So, you haven't seen this before?"

"Well, mental health is not an exact science, Pat." He closed the book. "But no, I haven't. I see many patients that are bipolar. And that's how I'd suggest we treat this. We're going to increase the Seroquel dramatically. We'll continue using the Ativan and Restoril, that won't change."

"So, you think Mia just needed more Seroquel, and she wouldn't have had the relapse?" I asked, hopeful that he might have solved our problem.

"Seroquel is in a group of medications called atypical antipsychotics. You don't really need to know that, but what you do need to know is that these drugs work by balancing the levels of neurotransmitters in the brain, increasing the amount of serotonin while dampening the amount of dopamine." He could tell that I was still waiting for an answer. "I'm not sure if we could have prevented a relapse, as you say, but I do believe that with an increased level of Seroquel your wife's thinking will return to normal."

"Great," I said, but something was still troubling me. "Dr. Martinez, the psychiatrist we saw in the emergency room, he thought she was suffering from brief reactive psychosis. That's a onetime event. Bipolar sounds more serious."

"We don't know what we're dealing with here," he responded. "Let's not worry about that right now. Let's get the psychosis under control. It could be a lot of things."

"And how long do you think that will take, to get it under control?" I asked, thinking of the last twenty-four hours and wondering how much more I could handle.

"With medication, almost all cases of psychosis resolve in four to eight days."

I contemplated another week. It was difficult to imagine, but I didn't have a choice.

"Okay." I nodded. "Okay, we can do that."

"Good." He handed me a prescription. "I can't take her up to six hundred milligrams immediately. We'll scale it up over the next few days. See my directions. And let's keep your appointment for Monday. Hopefully, things will have improved by then."

He said it so optimistically, and he seemed so knowledgeable, that it gave me confidence.

I only had to survive the weekend.

7.

THE PLAN

Beastie Boys and Miho Hatori
"I Don't Know"
1:49–2:17

Mia never gave up on helping me find the cause of my illness. "We need to keep looking," she would say as we'd bundle up to make yet another trip to the research library at the University of Chicago.

I had been sick for two years when I started having additional aches in my joints. Mia suggested seeing a specialist in rheumatoid arthritis. "It causes the kind of joint problems that you're describing. I've never heard of it being associated with abdominal pain, but I guess it's possible."

When we saw the specialist, he disagreed with her. "No, you don't have rheumatism," he told us, "but it could be autoimmune related, maybe linked to some type of bowel disease." This was the break we needed.

A few months later, a colonoscopy showed clear signs of Crohn's disease. Neither Mia nor I knew much about it, but we quickly became experts. The disease had no known cause or cure. It was an autoimmune disorder in which the body attacked the small and large intestines, causing inflammation and pain. Another common indication was severe diarrhea, which fortunately I did not have. My abnormal presentation of symptoms was the reason it took so long to find the correct diagnosis.

I was relieved to finally have an answer, but it was a devastating one. The doctor delivered a crushing prognosis: "Pat, you must learn to live with pain. We might be able to help things with medication, but you have a chronic disease. It isn't going away."

Thankfully, Mia kept me from losing hope. Several months later, we stumbled across a little-known book called *Breaking the Vicious Cycle* by Elaine Gottschall. The author outlines her thesis that Crohn's disease is caused by an imbalance of the bacterial colonies lining the intestines. She also introduces a diet designed to reestablish balance, eradicate the pain, and restore health.

The diet is unbelievably strict: no gluten, lactose, or refined sugar. You aren't supposed to eat anything that you haven't prepared yourself; you have to be certain of the ingredients. It is a difficult regimen to follow and would require huge investments of time.

Fortunately, I had Mia's support. She helped me start the diet and stick to it. We embraced all the cooking that had to be done. Back then, you couldn't find gluten-free options like you can today. We spent our weekends buying whole almonds and grinding them into flour or making shaved zucchini into pizza dough. Some of the recipes were really wacky.

But the diet worked! Slowly but surely, my intestines began to heal, and the pain subsided. Within five years, I was completely healthy again. It was truly a miracle, and it wouldn't have been possible without Mia's encouragement and hands-on help.

When you are sick, and the experts don't have any answers, you need an advocate. You need someone who believes in you, who will stick by your side and never give up.

I shudder to think what would have happened to me without Mia's support.

***

On the way home from the appointment, we stopped at the pharmacy to pick up the new prescription. Mia was moving from twenty-five-milligram tablets of Seroquel to one-hundred-milligram pills. Stronger doses made me nervous, but I was reassured by Dr. Martinez's promise that higher levels of the psychotropic drug would address her psychosis.

We started increasing the medication on Friday afternoon, but that evening was similar to the previous night. Mia did her best to stay quiet during dinner, and I did my best to have patience with her while we were holed up in our bedroom. It wasn't ideal, but it was tolerable.

When Mia fell asleep, I spoke with her cousin Alex again, interested in his view as a psychiatrist. He agreed with Dr. Martinez's recommendation to increase the Seroquel dosage. When I told him that she would be taking six hundred milligrams of Seroquel daily along with the Ativan and Restoril, his response was memorable: "Pat, that amount of medication would make a three-hundred-pound man sleep for three days."

Laughing, I made a comment about not minding if Mia slept that long, but the humor masked a grave concern.

How severe was her brain imbalance that even with all that medication she was only sleeping six hours a night? "Alex, I'm really worried," I confided. "This has to work. All I want is for her to get better, but I don't know what to do."

"You're doing everything you can," he assured me. "Let the medicine do its job. Even though Mia's sick now, she knows you're with her. Trust me, that means everything, even if she can't express it."

The following morning, I sensed a change in her behavior. Mia was becoming less fixated on the details of the past week and more concerned with the broader picture. At times, she had moments of self-awareness. "Oh my God, Pat, what is happening to me?" she asked repeatedly, her eyebrows pulled together in worry. But then, moments later, she was lost again.

We now had a calendar with detailed notes scrawled across every day in September. We also had my small notebook, in which I had logged comments from Mark, Dr. Patel, and Alex, along with the recent addition of Dr. Martinez's instructions. Periodically, Mia would review them with determined concentration, as if attempting to solve a crossword puzzle without any clues.

"Something is going on, Pat, what is it?" she would ask every ten minutes or so.

"You and I are spending time together," I began replying, stripping all emotion from my response. "Dr. Martinez gave us a plan, and we are following the plan." Then, I would pull out my notebook. While we were in his office, I had scribbled:

The Plan:
600 milligrams Seroquel

Ativan the same
Restoril the same
4-8 days

Each time this happened, Mia grabbed the notebook and recited "*The Plan*" out loud to herself. She must have read it thirty times that morning. "I'm glad we have the plan," she would say, sighing, and then revert to her psychotic behavior.

Around midday, she became fixated on going back in time again, much like she had in Celia's garage.

"Pat, we need to start going backward," she demanded continuously, as if her survival depended on it. "We need to play it back. If we play it backward, everything will be okay."

She acted as if I could make it happen. Feeling helpless, I kept refocusing her attention on Dr. Martinez's instructions. "No, that isn't the plan," I would respond, flat toned. "Dr. Martinez gave us a plan, and we are sticking to the plan."

"Right, right, the plan," she would repeat, taking the notebook from me.

As the day drew on, more paranoia began to creep into her deliberations. At various points, she became convinced that our room was being bugged or secretly videotaped. She also started talking about the devil again, like she had in Mark's truck. She was working through a theory that Satan could travel between people when they looked at each other, jumping from one brain to the other through direct line of sight.

Surprising, Mia's behavior wasn't obviously deranged. If you had a machine that could analyze body language and vocal intonations, without focusing on her words or the meaning of her sentences, you probably wouldn't have noticed anything wrong. She looked normal; her voice sounded normal. And this made our interactions that much more disturbing, especially all the talk about Satan. She described her theory regarding the devil like she would any other scientific hypothesis.

She never once questioned staying in the bedroom. It was as if she knew that isolation was better than being around other people.

When we finally emerged for dinner on Saturday night, I was physically and mentally exhausted. I hadn't slept much in a week, using the time that Mia was asleep to update the family and catch up on work. My patience was wearing thin, too. Being around a psychotic person nonstop was becoming unbearable.

Additionally, I was concerned about the kids; we hadn't spent much time together in a week. On Sunday morning, I decided to escape the house with them. We needed a break, and Mia's parents could watch her while I was gone.

After a few hours of visiting parks, smiles had replaced the serious faces that had started the day. When we were back in the car to return home, I took the opportunity to ask how they were doing. Will seemed fine, but Jamie was quiet, which was rare for her. I sensed that something was wrong, so I pressed harder.

She looked at me uneasily. "I know you're busy, and this isn't that important," she said, "but I'm just sad that I missed my tea party yesterday."

Her sentence hit me like a shock. For months, she had been looking forward to that party. Her Girl Scouts troop was holding it at a high-end British restaurant, complete with crumpets and jam.

"Oh, Jamie," I said, with a guilt-racked conscience, "I wish you would have reminded me! I feel terrible!"

"I don't want you to feel terrible, Daddy," she said. "I wasn't going to tell you, but you kept asking. I was just being honest."

"I'm glad you told me," I said, "but I'm so mad at myself. I should have taken you."

"No, it's okay, it's not that important," she repeated, and for some reason that made me feel even worse. I heard it like, "It's okay, *I'm* not that important."

"No," I said, "it's not okay, Jamie. You are just as important as everyone else in this family. I will make it up to you. We'll go to tea together, okay? We'll do it this week. I promise."

Of course, I had no idea how I would find time to take Jamie to tea. I hadn't really been to the office in a week, and Mia required so much of my attention. Even so, the kids needed my support, too. I was painfully aware that the situation could cause serious harm to their emotional development, and I was determined not to let it. I knew that Mia would want me to prioritize the kids, too.

Walking back into the house, any thought of the kids quickly evaporated. I was appalled to see Mia sitting on the couch across from Marcos, instructing him on some kind of experiment. He was holding his hand over his left eye.

"Right, now look straight into my right eye," Mia commanded. "No, you have to cover your left eye completely, or the results will not be accurate. Any obstacle could interfere with the transfer of thought."

"Oh, sorry," he said, moving his hand higher in deep concentration. They were seated about two feet away from each other. Mia had a pad of paper beside her, acting like a scientist conducting research.

Maybe it was my lack of sleep, but I found the entire scene incredibly upsetting. I couldn't believe that he was playing along with her delusions, although I shouldn't have been surprised. From experience, I knew how difficult it was to interact with Mia in her current state. You didn't know if you should try to talk sense into her, ignore her, or pretend that she was acting normally.

Playing along seemed the worst approach to me. I thought it would encourage her psychosis, egging her on to wilder ideas. I rushed over to the couch, breaking them up, and quickly ushered Mia back into our room.

She was going on about her new theory. It was something about the power of the eyes and how ideas could be transferred from one person to another through vision. It was eerily similar to her devil-speak from the previous day, only her arguments were becoming more and more spirited, like she was sliding deeper into psychosis.

I became increasingly distraught, blaming myself for leaving her with her parents, but that didn't have anything to do with it. Her behavior was changing because the Seroquel levels in her body were steadily rising. Still, I decided not to ask Marcos and Lucia to watch her again.

I called my mom to see if she and my stepdad could visit for a while. She immediately agreed, although they couldn't make it to our house until Tuesday. Fortunately, Celia had recently texted, wanting to know if she could help. I responded to her message and asked if she could come until my mom arrived. Not only would Celia provide backup support if needed, but her visit would be good for the kids. She could be loud, but she was funny. And at that point, we all needed a laugh.

Celia pulled into the driveway a few hours later, right as we were sitting down for dinner. After greeting everyone, she pulled me aside. "Oh my God, Pat!" she cried. "You look terrible. Have you slept at all?"

"Not really," I admitted. "I'm averaging about four hours a night."

"It's not enough. You need to get sleep. What good will it do Mia or the kids if you get yourself sick? I can stay with her tonight."

"Celia, it's pretty tough. You spent time with her last Sunday. Remember how uncomfortable you were? I have more experience with it now."

"I can do it, Pat," she assured me. "You need to rest."

The thought of a full night's sleep was mesmerizing, but I already felt guilty for having left Mia that morning. Still, I knew Celia was right. I reluctantly acquiesced and gave her the night shift.

Will and Jamie were thrilled when they heard that I would be spending the rest of the night with them. "You can sleep in my bed tonight, Daddy," Jamie offered. "You're so tired, and you'll sleep better that way."

"Yeah," chimed in Will, "and I'll give you my extra pillow!"

"Right, and my stuffed animals!" echoed Jamie.

"And we'll read to you for a change," added Will.

They had fun going back and forth, coming up with ways to pamper me. It turned into a memorable event, and I relished every second. It was such a relaxing change from the unrelenting stress of being around Mia. They treated me like the child, tucking me in, hugging me good night, and turning out the lights as they snuck out of the room. I fell asleep as soon as they left.

I woke feeling rejuvenated from my first full night's sleep in over a week. Celia was frazzled, informing me that she and Mia had been up early. I offered to take over. Mia and I were scheduled to see Dr. Martinez later that day, and I wanted to get a sense of her condition.

It became immediately clear that Mia was not responding to the medication. Her anxiety levels were even higher than the day before. She was raving about Mensa, an organization for people with high IQs. She was convinced that some of our relatives were members, and she wanted to know what secrets they were keeping from us.

Mia was also still obsessing over her theory concerning eyesight, having remembered Satan's role in her hypothesis. She broached the idea that the devil had been in her dad's brain while they were conducting their experiments the prior day. She was trying to figure out if Satan had escaped during their experiments and might be lurking in close proximity. This last detail was alarming. Mia had been talking about the devil off and on for a week, but this was the first time she mentioned him being in the house.

Even though I had pledged not to respond to her outlandish ideas, I felt compelled to quash these thoughts immediately. "No, Mia," I stated firmly, "the devil is not in our house." She abruptly stopped talking and gave me a suspicious look like, *How can you be so sure about that, Pat?* I ignored her, hoping that would be the end of it.

About midmorning, we started preparing for the doctor's appointment. I was in the shower, and as the water rained down from the showerhead, I thought about Dr.

Martinez's plan. As I walked back into the bedroom, I was wondering what more he might recommend.

"Pat, we need to kill the dog," Mia said in a calm voice. She was standing by the foot of the bed, our old miniature dachshund cradled in her arms.

"What are you talking about?" I gasped. Chica was like our firstborn child. We had adopted her as a puppy right after our wedding, and Mia loved her as much as I did.

"It's the devil," she lamented. "He got inside her." I started to look down, but she cut me off. "Don't look into her eyes!" she shouted.

Oh right, I thought to myself, *because if I look into her eyes, Satan might jump into me.*

"Mia, sweetheart," I pleaded, "I know you are upset, but this is our little baby, remember? She's been with us for fourteen years. She's so sweet. We don't need to do anything to her." I was slowly taking our dog into my arms, careful not to look down. Mia seemed relieved. "Now, I am going to take her out of the room, and then you and I can review the plan, okay?"

"Okay," she said, absently walking over to sit on the bed.

We soon left for Dr. Martinez's office. As we sat in the waiting area, white noise humming in the background, I thought about the seventy-two hours since we had last seen him. According to the plan, the psychosis might be close to resolving. That seemed unlikely given the events of the morning.

After ushering us into his office, Dr. Martinez asked Mia a few questions. He quickly surmised by her answers and conduct that things hadn't changed. He turned to me instead. "Pat, how would you describe the last three days with Mia?"

I had to be careful. Although Mia might not be thinking straight, she would be listening. "Well, Doctor," I began, "she has been fairly agitated. It seems to be getting worse. This morning, she was convinced that the devil had possessed our dog. I assured her that this wasn't the case, and that we didn't need to kill Chica. But obviously, Mia is having a lot of trouble relaxing right now. She's frightened that Satan is hiding somewhere in our house."

"I see," replied Dr. Martinez, his eyes widening. "Okay, we are going to change the plan. We have increased her dose to six hundred milligrams of Seroquel. We are now going to move it up to eight hundred milligrams."

"What?" I choked out, louder than I would have liked. "With all due respect, Dr. Martinez, the increases in medication seem to be aggravating Mia's anxiety. Might we consider toning it down a little?"

"No, Pat," he responded. "Mia's thought disorder is not responding to the smaller dosage. We need to increase the medication and let time do its job." I gave him an uneasy look. "Trust me on this, Pat, Mia will come around. We need to get the acute phase of this under control. The medication is the way to do that."

Dr. Martinez stood up after scribbling his new instructions. "Here is the new dosage. Ativan and Restoril stay the same. Seroquel moves up to eight hundred milligrams per day immediately." He reached out his hand to shake mine. "See my assistant, and let's set up an appointment for Thursday."

He began to usher us out of his office. It seemed rushed, but maybe he didn't want to say a lot in front of Mia. I wondered how much of our exchange she had followed. She walked back into the waiting area, and I was starting to follow when Dr. Martinez pulled me aside.

"Pat," he said, his face grim, "I work closely with the Gulfshore Treatment Center." I had heard of the GTC. It was our local mental health facility. "In fact, I am the head psychiatrist for the crisis center there. The staff at the GTC, we have a lot of experience dealing with this kind of thing."

"I'm sure you do," I replied. I had never visited the GTC, nor did I know anyone who had been there. All I could think of was Mark's description of those places, and how determined he had been to keep Mia out of them.

"This is my personal cell phone number," he said, handing me a slip of paper. "If things get too difficult for you, call or text me. I can get the team at the crisis center ready for Mia and make sure she is safe."

I stood looking down at his number. "We'll be fine," I said, without much conviction.

"I appreciate what you are doing, but if you ever feel that Mia is a danger to herself or to others, you need to get help. What you said here today was very concerning."

"I know, but it's only another day or so."

"Hopefully, but remember, this can sometimes take over a week to work itself out."

"I don't want to take her to a mental facility. She's better off at home."

"She's better off safe," he said firmly, "and so are you, Pat. Please, if you need help, call me."

All the way home I kept thinking about what he had said, about Mia becoming a danger. It didn't seem possible, but the whole thing with Chica that morning had been creepy. Maybe he had a point. And it was imperative to keep Mia safe; I did agree with that.

Celia was waiting for us when we walked into the house. I could tell that she was still rattled from the previous night. After getting Mia settled back into our room, I ducked out quickly to speak with Celia alone.

"Could you do me a favor," I asked, "and help with the kids when they get home from school? I think they could do with a change of pace, and you're so good with them."

I could see the relief on Celia's face. "Yeah, sure, I'd love to spend time with Will and Jamie," she said. She paused, and then with a frown continued. "It's so upsetting, seeing Mia like this."

"I know."

"If anyone in our family was going to go through something like this, I would have bet on me. Hell, Pat, everyone would have bet on me. But Mia? Never. I still can't believe this is happening to her."

"I can't believe it, either. But we'll get her back, Celia, I can promise you that."

But as the day wore on, I knew we weren't getting her back anytime soon. Mia's paranoia was as severe as it had been earlier in the day. Our conversation rambled through many of the same disturbing tirades: Mensa, messages from God, the truth, the plan, the devil.

Watching over Mia that night was arduous. She had more energy, and as her energy increased, so did my anxiety levels. Plus, all the talk about the devil had gone from spooky to spine chilling, like she could sense him lurking in the shadows of our room. And her thoughts were racing so dramatically that her mood could turn in an instant.

With reluctance, I began increasing her Seroquel dose yet again. I had mixed feelings about it. Her psychosis was getting worse, that seemed obvious. But according to Dr. Martinez, this was the only way to get it under control.

As soon as Mia fell asleep, I crept to our back room, fatigued and apprehensive. I needed some quiet time before trying to fall asleep.

I opened my email. Along with a slew of work-related messages, I also received a note from my brother, Brad. He was supportive and optimistic, promising that Mia would recover. Smiling tearfully, I agreed, confessing that I couldn't bear to think otherwise.

Climbing back into bed next to her, for a moment I sat studying Mia. She remained as beautiful as ever, with that serene look on her face that accompanies sleep. For what seemed like the millionth time, I wondered what was happening inside her brain. I downloaded a book on bipolar disorder and started reading, but I stopped after twenty minutes. Dr. Martinez was right; it didn't fit.

Lying silently in the dark, I reflected on Brad's positive message. Sooner or later, the medication would start working, and my lovely wife would return. Life had confronted us with a major obstacle, but what mattered was how we responded. I was a fighter, and I knew that Mia was, too.

I fell asleep confident that I could handle whatever the illness threw at me the following day.

8.

THE DEVIL

The Killers
"A Dustland Fairytale"
0:44–0:58

One day during our second winter in Chicago, I came home from work complaining about the frigid temperature. "You know," Mia pointed out, "there are places we could live where it stays warm all year round." As much as I loved the Midwest, her comment stuck, and later that spring I accepted a position with a company in Houston.

The timing was right. My investment banking job was a two-year commitment, and it was coming to an end. Mia was finishing her first year in the physician assistant master's program at the University of North Chicago. Her second year would consist of six-week rotations at various hospitals and doctors' offices. These internships could be located anywhere across the country.

Finally, after completing several rotations away, she moved to one of her Houston-based assignments. We were excited to be together again, and she lived in my apartment on the outskirts of the city. Mia worked downtown, though, and the drive was an hour each way. In addition, her rotation was in the emergency room at Ben Taub Hospital. She had twelve-hour shifts in one of the busiest medical centers in Texas. The lack of sleep and long commute were challenges.

If she had the night shift, we wouldn't see each other until right before I left for work. But one morning, she didn't return home at her usual time. I waited an extra thirty minutes before finally leaving. Those were the days before cell phones, so I stuck a note on the counter asking her to call as soon as possible.

"Sorry, babe," she said after I jumped to answer the phone a couple of hours later. "My shift ran over last night, and I was so tired, I couldn't make the drive home."

"Are you okay? Where are you now?"

"Yeah, don't worry, I'm home now," she said quickly. But I remained concerned as she told me about locking her doors and sleeping in her car. In a poorly lit parking garage. In downtown Houston.

My life as a banker had been sleep deprived, but Mia was managing a far worse schedule than I ever had.

Another issue with the rotation was the stress. Ben Taub was a Level 1 trauma center, which meant that the most extreme cases were sent to its emergency room. Mia saw all kinds of nasty stuff during her time there: homicides, car accidents, drug overdoses. Confident in her ability to save lives, Mia tackled the job with determination and vigor.

Frequently, she would want to talk about the various crises she had faced. Not the specifics of the patients—she couldn't do that—but what she had seen and learned. But the blood-and-guts stuff didn't sit well with me. I never wanted to listen, and she knew it.

However, I did hear about one event. She came home from a night shift visibly more shaken than normal. "Do you want to talk about it?" I asked, pulling her close. It was a testament to the seriousness of the situation that she accepted my offer.

"We were so busy last night." She wasn't crying; she sounded emotional but composed. "Everyone was running in a million directions.

"A teenager came into the ER. Her parents brought her in. Pat, she had tried to commit suicide. Both of her wrists had been slashed. Her mom was holding towels to her arms, but there was blood everywhere."

"Good Lord," I whispered.

"A few car accidents had just come in." She sounded far away, as if she were reliving the shock from a safe distance. "No one else was free, so she was assigned to me. I didn't even have a doctor to consult with."

I didn't know what to say.

"I stitched up both of her wrists. She just sat there looking down at her arms while I did it."

My wife could handle extreme stress. One didn't survive the horror of the Ben Taub emergency room without being able to manage pressure. And she could go without sleep, too. I'd seen her do it for weeks.

So, had stress from her work and a lack of sleep triggered Mia's psychosis? All the doctors thought so. But why didn't any issues arise when the sleep deprivation and work trauma were levels of magnitude greater?

***

Tuesday began early. Immediately, it became clear that Mia was as anxious and paranoid as the night before. I resigned myself to the fight, accepting that we wouldn't be taming the illness on the short end of Dr. Martinez's range of four to eight days.

Mia had moments of surprising clarity that morning. She would be talking about some disconnected idea and then suddenly switch topics. "Oh my God, Pat!" she would cry. "Something is wrong with me! We have to go backward, or else I'll have to go to the treatment center!"

She couldn't have heard Dr. Martinez speaking about it, so she must have known about the GTC through her job. She mentioned it several times. I had no answers when she did. I kept trying to redirect her to the plan, but she had lost all interest in it.

Her mood was vacillating so wildly that it was becoming more difficult to influence her. I resorted to remaining as calm and unexpressive as possible, hoping that my stillness might counteract her high energy.

Marcos and Lucia went to the store midmorning. At about the same time, Mia became focused on leaving the bedroom.

"I need to get out of here," she kept saying, as if in warning. She was talking to herself, her eyes darting from the windows to the doors. "I can't stay here." She revisited the idea every five minutes, looping it around with her other racing thoughts.

She was clearly plotting some kind of escape. She had stopped looking at me when speaking. It started gradually and then became evident. She would turn her head in the other direction or stare at the floor. Even if I addressed her directly, she would avoid my gaze.

Mia never accused me of becoming the devil, but her actions made it clear. She couldn't look into my eyes because then Satan himself would have a direct link into her brain. She was slowly moving physically farther away from me, too, hoping that I wouldn't notice. Mia was acting like someone in a murder mystery who has finally solved the crime but doesn't want the culprit to know.

It must have been terrifying for her. For the past week, I had been the one person she could trust through her fog of paranoia. But then, suddenly, I was compromised, taken over by a demon from her nightmares. Attempting to keep her in our room seemed like an especially bad idea.

Reluctantly, I decided to let her go, knowing that Celia was home and the house was locked. I pretended to use the bathroom and left Mia alone for a few minutes. Sure enough, when I came back, the bedroom door was open and she had gone.

I stood still for a moment, scanning the empty room and thinking about the kids. What would happen if they returned from school to find their mom running away from their dad, screaming that he was possessed by the devil?

Slowly walking into the hallway, I was at a loss for what to do. Celia found me in a dazed kind of stupor, staring blankly ahead. "Is everything okay?" she asked. "Where's Mia?"

"She's in the house somewhere," I whispered. "You know how the devil has been bouncing around recently?"

"Yeah?"

"Well, as of about twenty minutes ago, he bounced into me."

Her eyebrows flew up over panicked eyes. "Pat, what are we going to do?"

I was already reaching into my pocket for Dr. Martinez's number. "The psychiatrist told me to call if I needed his advice." I said it calmly and slowly, trying to keep my emotions in check. "I need it now."

Dr. Martinez answered quickly. I was explaining how Mia believed me to be possessed, when something started clanging in the backyard.

Celia and I whipped our heads around. Mia was standing at the back of our lanai, a screened-in area surrounding the pool, trying desperately to open the door to the backyard. She was yanking the handle, slamming it repeatedly against the screen enclosure. Without thinking, I raced out to stop her.

"Mia," I asked, skidding to a halt, "what are you doing?" I tried to sound composed. Refusing to look at me, she frantically continued tugging on the door. It was like a scene from a horror movie, where the victim tries to flee as the monster approaches. It was surreal to feel like the monster. Fortunately, I had bolted the door when Mia's psychosis had returned, and she'd forgotten it had a lock.

"Babe," I repeated, "are you going somewhere?"

"Stay away from me, Pat!" she shouted. "I'm going to visit the neighbors! You can't stop me!"

I had the distinct impression that Mia was not going next door; she was trying to get as far away from me as possible. Fortunately, Celia had followed me out. "But Mia," I said softly, "your sister is here to visit you. Why don't you spend time with her?"

Celia took the cue perfectly. "Yeah, come into the house with me," she said, moving toward Mia as I stepped to the side. "You get to see your neighbors all the time. Let's go talk." She put her arm around Mia and started coaxing her away from the door. Not looking in my direction, Mia moved uncertainly back inside.

I remembered the phone. "Dr. Martinez?"

"Yes, I'm here," he responded. "Is everything okay?"

"No," I confessed in fear. "Mia was trying to escape our backyard. I think she was running away."

I heard him let out a breath. "Look, Pat," he said, "it's your decision, but I strongly advise you to bring Mia into the treatment center. I can meet you when you arrive."

He was right. What would have happened if Mia had run away? "Okay, we'll leave right away."

He gave me directions, but I was only half listening. Instead, I was trying to rationalize sending Mia to a mental health facility after Mark had fought so heroically to keep her out.

After shoving a couple of Mia's sweats and T-shirts into a duffel bag, I grabbed my car keys. I could hear Celia talking to Mia in the living room. "Celia!" I called from the hallway. "Let's go for a car ride. Bring Mia along. I'll drive."

Celia didn't know where we were headed, but she followed my lead. "Come on," she said with encouragement, leading Mia to the garage. "It'll be good to get out of the house."

Mia appeared hesitant, but she was going along with it. Climbing into the back seat, she abruptly became angry again. "Where are we going, Pat?" she began demanding. "What are you planning to do with us, Pat?!"

I sat in the driver's seat with the engine running and the air conditioner blasting. I kept my eyes straight ahead and pretended that I was oblivious to Mia's barrage of questions. My hands were shaking; my only focus was getting to the facility as fast as possible.

We started driving. Mia was speaking to herself loudly, having given up on any response from me. She was trying to determine our destination by the route we were taking. "We're going to the Gulfshore Treatment Center," she proclaimed. "I knew it!"

But then I missed a turn. My system was flooded with adrenaline, perspiration dripping down my forehead. It was hard to keep focus. "The treatment center was that way!" exclaimed Mia, looking behind us. "Where are you taking us now? Where are we going?" She sounded less triumphant and more scared.

Poor Celia—she had no idea what was going on. I was completely silent, still not daring to acknowledge the truth. Mia sounded like a detective trying to reason through a case when none of the clues were making sense. She kept muttering things like, "Are we going to the high school? Why would he be taking us to the high school?"

Finally, I recovered the correct route, and Mia quickly zeroed in on the right answer again. "We *are* going to the treatment center!" Soon we were pulling into the main driveway.

The Gulfshore Treatment Center occupied a small site on the outskirts of Sarasota. The campus comprised several single-story stucco buildings, all painted a drab yellow color. They didn't have many windows, and I imagined that the interiors were dark and private. Overgrown oak trees hid most of the area's perimeter, and palm trees filled the open spaces between buildings.

Signs for the crisis center led us to the back of the campus. As we drove around the buildings, I saw Dr. Martinez and another woman waiting. I swung the car into the drop-off area, and Celia opened the back door. She and Mia were whisked quickly inside.

"Welcome to my other office," Dr. Martinez said. "I was hoping not to see you here."

"Yeah, me too. What happens next?"

"That's it, Pat, at least for now. We take it from here."

"But I'd like to see Mia. I want to make sure she's okay."

"She'll be okay," he promised. "I'm the head psychiatrist here at the center. She'll be under my care and that of the other doctors here."

"Okay," I said, "but I'd still like to see her. I want to make sure she knows that I'm here for her."

"Of course," he replied with a slight grimace. "But right now, aren't you here because she didn't want to see you?"

"Yes." It was a simple answer to a complicated question.

"Pat, there's something you should know, if you don't already," he said. "Mia is coming here of her own volition, but I am going to keep her until I feel she is ready to leave. It might be a few days; it might be a week. We'll see how she does. I have that authority."

"I know. It's called the Baker Act."

"Correct," he confirmed, "but the other thing you should know is that you can only see Mia if and when she wants to see you. You can only talk to her if she wants to talk to you."

"What?" I was surprised. "No, I don't like that. It's important for me to be with her. She needs to know I'm here." I was having second thoughts. Although I liked Dr. Martinez, I hadn't even seen what the facility looked like.

"I understand. Come with me. Maybe we can catch her while they're in admitting." We stepped inside the entrance and into a small lobby. It was barren and bleak. There was a receptionist window straight ahead, a few chairs against the walls, and a single door off to the right.

Dr. Martinez approached the door and glanced at the receptionist, his fingers around the handle. A buzzer sounded, and he pulled it open. Walking through, I saw that we had entered a short hallway with a few doors on either side. I couldn't see the end of the corridor; it turned after about a dozen feet. Dr. Martinez gestured to the first door on the left.

"She'll be in there," he said. "I'll wait here."

Entering a small office, I saw Mia and Celia sitting at a desk, across from the woman who had been at the entrance. She was young, probably in her late twenties. Mia was taking off her rings and giving them to Celia.

"I don't want him in here!" Mia said, eyeing me angrily. "He needs to leave!" She was addressing the young woman, who had looked up from some papers on the desk. The woman gave me a compassionate smile. Celia appeared completely helpless.

"GET OUT OF HERE, PAT!!" screamed Mia, glaring at me.

Startled, I took a step backward. "I'll wait outside," I mumbled. "Mia, I'll be right here if you need me." That last bit made no sense, given the circumstances.

Dr. Martinez remained standing in the hallway. He gave me a sympathetic pat on the shoulder and ushered me back into the lobby.

"Visiting hours are six to eight in the evening, noon to two during the day," he said. "When you come, you'll check in at the window. But remember, Pat, you can only go back if Mia approves your visit."

"Right," I responded, but my mind was reliving the moment when Mia had screamed at me.

"Also," Dr. Martinez added, "the center doesn't allow children under thirteen to visit. It's too hard on them. I hope you understand."

I nodded despondently. He excused himself, informing me that he had to check on Mia's status.

It took a few minutes to start processing thoughts again. Pulling out my phone, I sent a group text. I wanted at least Mark, Brad, my mom, and Mia's parents to know what had happened:

> Mia thought the devil was in me today
> She tried to run away
> Her doctor strongly advised me to bring
> her to the mental health facility
> That's where she is now
> At least she is safe

Immediately, two texts came in reply:

> *Mark:* You did what you had to do, it was
> the right thing

> *Brad:* I'm so sorry, let us know what we
> can do

I didn't want to respond. All I wanted was Mia back, the person I had fallen in love with. But the illness had taken her hostage, and now I had no legal right to even see her.

The ride home was eerily quiet, like being in the eye of a hurricane. The calm stillness was such a contrast to the frantic mood of everything prior.

"I can't believe that just happened," I admitted finally, sighing in defeat.

"Neither can I," groaned Celia. She turned to me. "Pat, you had to do it. You didn't have a choice."

"Guess so," I said half-heartedly, still not convinced it was the right decision. "Thanks for being there with me, Celia. I know it wasn't easy."

"I don't know how you did it as long as you did," she replied. "I only spent one night with her, and that was horrible."

I couldn't talk; opening my mouth would only result in tears. Celia was looking at me, but she must have seen my eyes watering. She faced forward again, and we passed the rest of the trip in silence.

Marcos and Lucia had returned while we were out. They both gave me long embraces. "Oh, Pat," whispered Lucia, her voice soft in my ear, "this is the best thing for Mia."

I nodded. It felt like I was swimming through a hazy dream, trying to keep my head above water. Marcos said nothing while he hugged me, but I could feel the teardrops on his cheeks. I struggled, fighting hard to keep my own emotions in check.

But at that moment our front door opened, and I saw my mom and stepdad coming into the house. We have always shared a close relationship, my mom and I. When I was growing up, she was the kind of parent who constantly gave her kids the benefit of the doubt. She trusted and supported us, and she was always a great comfort to me in times of need. Seeing her that day, I was instantly ten years old again.

My mom didn't hesitate. She walked directly over without saying a word and wrapped her arms around me. And then I lost it. Ten days of worries, fears, false hopes, and failures came pouring out. I was suddenly crying and shaking, sucking in great gulps of air.

"There was nothing I could do," I sobbed. "All I wanted was to help her get better."

"I know, I know," my mom whispered in my ear.

"I thought that if I could stay with her, if I could just be patient, that my love would make the sickness go away."

"I know, I know."

"But nothing I did mattered. It just kept getting worse."

"Patrick, honey, you did everything you could," my mom reassured me. She kept repeating it, as if doing so would rid me of all doubt. "You did everything you could."

But had I done everything I could? I didn't know. I had never dealt with mental illness before. It was difficult to predict and disconcerting; at times, it was downright scary. Plus, the tools at my disposal were inaccurate at best. We were feeding Mia all kinds of medications without much knowledge of exactly how they worked.

My mom and I stood in that embrace for a long time, much longer than a normal hug. As the emotion drained from my fatigued body, I began to compose myself. By the time Marcos and Lucia left our house, my tears had dried. I was fully collected when Celia drove away, making me promise that I would keep her updated.

Will and Jamie were excited to see their grandparents when they came home from school. I gave them time together before sitting the kids down for an update.

I collected myself and tried to look confident. Again, the right words were hard to find.

"Okay, you know how Mom has been sick?" They both nodded, becoming suddenly very serious. "Well, like we talked about before, sometimes when people get sick, we might think that they're better, but they can still have some of the sickness left inside."

Two concerned stares. Worried eyes.

"And sometimes, if there is a lot of sickness left inside, they can have to go back to the hospital. We call it a relapse. And what it means is that they just need more time with the doctors. But that's all they need, more time. And then they're going to get better."

Silence.

"Mom had to go back to the hospital today. Not the same hospital, not the one where Uncle Mark works. But a different hospital, one here in Sarasota. It's where people go if they have a sickness in their brain, and the doctors there have special training to help them.

"Now, I'm sure you are worried. So I'm going to let you ask me any questions that you have. I promise to answer them truthfully." I figured this was the best approach. I didn't want to start guessing how much detail to provide.

I sat on the floor, watching them. Jamie was perched on her bed, gazing down; Will was on the carpet a few feet away. They were both inspecting me, trying to read my body language.

Several seconds ticked by. Jamie was the first to speak. "Is Mommy going to die?"

"Oh no, Mommy's not going to die," I said, standing and scooping her into a hug. "Mommy is just sick, that's all, but I promise you that she's going to get better."

Jamie put her head against my shoulder. "Okay, Daddy, I believe you," she said, relaxing into my arms. Will remained on the floor, watching me.

"Will, how about you?" I asked. "What questions do you have?"

He sat very still, first looking at me and then down at his hands. After a pause, he said, without glancing up, "I want to see where she is."

"You want to see where she is?" I repeated, making sure I had it right. "You mean you want to see the building that she's in?"

"Yes, I want to see where she is." He didn't raise his head; he was studying his fingers.

"Okay, yes, we can do that. Unfortunately, we can't go inside and see her. It's not like a normal hospital; they have lots of restrictions about getting in. But yeah, we can jump in the car right now, and I can show you the building."

Jamie stayed with my parents while Will and I drove in silence to the treatment center. Once we had parked, I pointed to the crisis center. "She's just inside that door and down a hallway. Doctors and specialists are making sure she's okay."

Will studied the building. He looked like someone taking a memory test, where you are shown a picture briefly and then asked to describe it in detail.

After a couple of quiet minutes, he turned away. "Okay, we can go," he said softly.

He didn't say anything else during the ride home, and neither did I.

9

THE CRISIS CENTER

Modest Mouse
"Ocean Breathes Salty"
0:40–0:58

Mia and I never fought. In fact, we didn't have even a minor quarrel until a couple of years into our relationship. It was over the holidays. I was staying with my parents at a hotel in Miami, but they checked out a day before I was set to leave. Mia was furious that her parents hadn't invited me to spend the extra night with them.

The Delgados were staying at Mia's grandma's house. Her grandma lived next door to Mia's aunt, who lived in a kind of double house with Mia's uncle's sister. Another aunt and uncle lived in close proximity. Privacy was limited; Cuban relatives were everywhere.

"It's fine, babe," I said, dropping my bags onto the floor of a cheap motel room. "Your parents don't really know me yet, and the house over there is packed with people."

"Well, you could sleep on the couch then."

"C'mon, I'm sure your dad doesn't want us sleeping under the same roof."

"Why are you taking his side of this?" she snapped uncharacteristically.

"I'm not taking his side," I said, and then corrected myself. "Well, I guess I am taking his side. But it's fine." I moved to give her a hug.

"It's not fine." She hugged me back, but then quickly broke it off and grabbed my luggage. "It's not fine, and it's not going to happen."

I rolled my eyes. "Mia, don't." I tugged the bags out of her hands. "Look, I don't want to push it with your folks. We can survive one more night apart."

"I know, but making you sleep here seems so wrong," she grumbled. "Ugh, my parents! I don't understand them sometimes. I really don't!"

"Well, you're not going to change them tonight."

She gave a frustrated sigh and rushed out the door. It wasn't our usual goodbye, but I didn't think much of it.

Twenty minutes later, the phone in my room started ringing. When I picked up, Mia was on the line. "I'm sorry. I shouldn't have left you like I did."

"Oh no, babe, it's okay," I said. "You seemed a little upset, but I didn't take offense."

"No, I got short with you, and I shouldn't have. It's just my parents. They can really get to me."

She didn't have much need to apologize. As far as I could tell, her parents were about the only people for whom Mia had no patience. For everyone else, she had endless amounts of sympathy.

The thought of Mia yelling and threatening someone was beyond consideration. It would never happen.

***

Shortly after driving Will home, I returned to the treatment center for visiting hours. The receptionist looked up as I approached.

"Hi, I'm here to see Mia Dylan."

"Please sign your name on the list and take a seat," she said. "I'll let the staff know you are here. Someone will come and get you when your visit has been accepted."

The lobby was the size of a typical medical waiting room, although it didn't offer magazines or a television for passing the time. Except for the chairs, the place was empty. The walls were bare, too, and it was quiet. There were no windows.

Given that it was early, I didn't expect to be called right away. The chairs were those uncomfortable wooden ones, and I found myself sitting straight up with the back of my head leaning against the wall behind me, remembering the shell shock I had felt in the same spot earlier that day.

After ten minutes, an older woman came into the lobby. She checked in with the receptionist and took a seat against the opposite wall. Less than a minute later, the door that led back into the hallway opened, and her name was called.

Over the next several minutes, this happened two more times. People checked in and were called swiftly into the facility. And still I sat, waiting.

An hour later, as I was standing to stretch, I caught the eye of the receptionist. "Sorry," she offered.

I nodded slightly and gave her an acknowledging smile. *I know,* I thought sadly, *you can only let me back if my wife wants to see me.*

Eventually, I lost all hope of visiting Mia that night, but I couldn't bring myself to leave. If there was some chance, no matter how slim, that she might want to see me, I was going to be present for her.

The waiting gave me time to think. Mia handled so many of the kids' responsibilities. Missing Jamie's tea party was one mistake, but I couldn't let there be others. Will had golf, Jamie had Girl Scouts, and they both had dentists' visits, doctors' appointments, and countless other activities. Plus, I had to plan their breakfasts and lunches, not to mention our dinners. I couldn't ask grandparents to hang around forever, taking care of us. And then there was my job, which I hadn't really dealt with since Mia had become sick.

I used the last fifteen minutes of my wait to make a list of priorities for the coming few days. It was depressing to watch the people who had gained access come back through the lobby. They looked discouraged, but at least they had seen their loved ones.

At exactly 8:00 p.m. I stood, thanked the receptionist, and walked out. I tried to imagine what Mia was doing, but it was impossible. I had no idea what her surroundings looked like. I hoped that she felt safe and secure. At least she didn't have to worry that the devil was going to get her; she had left him waiting in the lobby.

I lay in bed for a long time that night, reveling in the newfound tranquility of our house. As relieved as I felt, I would have preferred having Mia back in the room with me. But she needed professional help, and at least at the GTC she would be receiving it.

The next morning, I went into work after the kids left for school. Fortunately, I had developed a close relationship with the wealthy family that had hired me a year earlier to help them manage their investments. Up to this point, all they knew was that Mia was sick and needed my care. Once again, the mental health stigma had kept me from being completely honest, but it was time to come clean.

Lori was the family member with whom I interacted most closely. She had studied psychology in college, and she had a relative who suffered from mental illness. She could immediately empathize with my situation. She told me to focus on Mia and implored me not to worry about work.

Even as the conversation was happening, I recognized how crucial it was. For most people, going through a severe mental health crisis would have meant financial hardship. Either that, or they would have had to sacrifice something to continue working, maybe support for their spouse or attention to their kids. What a privilege that my job could take lower priority, at least for a little while.

I left the office at lunchtime to return to the GTC for daytime visiting hours. Again, I checked in early and took a seat against the wall. The experience was identical to that of the night before. A few people came and were quickly called back while I waited, disappointed and helpless.

After sitting in silence for another two hours, I walked to my car in frustration. Mia knew I was in the lobby, yet she continued to shun me. Driving home, I tried to conceive of some way of convincing her to let me visit.

When the kids arrived home that afternoon, I suggested that we each make a card for their mom, telling her how much we loved her. "I'll draw her flowers because Mommy loves flowers!" exclaimed Jamie. "And you can draw her some of your stick figures, Will."

"No, I'll write her a poem," he replied. "It will be about how much I miss her. Maybe it will help her come back sooner."

Before long, we had paper, crayons, and colored pencils strewn across the kitchen table. I included a recent five-by-seven family portrait in my letter. Mia had loved the picture, and I hoped it would bring her comfort.

That evening was a replay of my last two visits. People signed in and were called back, and the receptionist continued to feel sorry for me. Periodically, I would stand up and stretch, being much less circumspect now that I was a regular. With five minutes left, I approached the window with our homemade cards.

"I'm sorry, Mr. Dylan," the receptionist lamented. "It's such a shame that we can't let you back."

"I know, I appreciate that. Say, can you do me a big favor?" I asked, putting the papers on the counter. "We made these for Mia. Can you please make sure that she gets them?"

The receptionist reached for our artwork, smiling. "Isn't that sweet? Yes, of course I can."

Back home, we enjoyed another calm night, but I was busy. My parents would be leaving soon, and I only had a few more days to plan for life after their departure.

At work the next day, I received a text from Will halfway through the morning:

> Dad, I'm worried
> I want to come home

He had never asked to come home from school before, not if he wasn't sick. I texted him back:

What do you mean, worried?
Mom is going to get better, Will

We hadn't spoken about our trip to the GTC, or about Mia's sickness, since our drive:

I know, I'm just worried
I want to come home

I wasn't sure what to do. My gut told me not to break down and pick him up:

I can't come and get you right now
Just get through the day and we'll talk about it after school
Sorry, my man, but everything will be okay

That was the last I heard from him, and I hoped that keeping him in school was the right call.

Once again, I left work before lunch and drove to the GTC. I desperately wanted to see if our handcrafted messages had influenced Mia. Apparently, they hadn't. She still refused to see me.

That afternoon, I walked to the end of our block to meet Will. He had been in my thoughts ever since our text exchange. When he stepped off the bus, I greeted him with a smile.

"Everything alright, Will?"

"I'm better now." He shrugged, letting me take his backpack. We started walking toward the house.

"Can you talk about it?" I asked.

"I don't know, Dad, I just started worrying and couldn't stop. It's like my thoughts were swirling around, and it just kept getting worse."

I was reminded of Mia's conversation with Alex; the "tornado of ideas" sounded eerily similar. I hoped that Will wasn't on the brink of his own mental health crisis.

"What were you worried about? Mom and everything going on?"

"No . . . yeah . . . I guess so. I don't know; I was just worried." He sounded frustrated, like he didn't want to talk about it.

I stopped walking and gave him a hug, wrapping him up like he was still a little kid. Most middle schoolers off the bus wouldn't have let me, but Will returned the embrace. "I know it's hard. It's hard for everyone, especially Mom." My voice wavered as I said the last part.

My mom and stepdad treated us to dinner that night. We went to a local Italian place, one of our favorites. The kids loved the chocolate cake, but I couldn't stay for dessert. I had to get back to the crisis center.

It was starting to feel like all I did was drive to the GTC. And wait, of course; I spent half my day waiting.

I was five minutes late for visiting hours. The receptionist offered me a sarcastic grin when I entered. "Mr. Dylan," she said, "for a minute, I thought maybe you'd given up."

"Never," I responded, returning the smile and taking my usual seat. After twenty minutes, I resigned myself to another eventless night. I took out my laptop and started working. But an hour later, the door into the facility opened.

"Pat Dylan?" a woman asked, and I looked up in disbelief.

"Yes?"

"Please follow me." She glanced down at my laptop. "But sir, you can't bring anything back."

"Oh right," I replied, quickly putting my computer in its bag. Standing up, I walked over to the receptionist. She looked as excited as I felt.

"Would you mind keeping an eye on this for me?" I handed her my pack.

"Of course," she said, smiling. "Good luck, Mr. Dylan."

"Thanks." I tried not to sound nervous. Flashing her a thumbs-up, I turned and followed the woman into the hallway.

As the corridor turned, I was surprised to see so much glass. A large window made up the top half of the left-hand side of the hallway. It looked into a big room, a kind of command center. I was reminded of those military movies where all the seats face a large computer screen. Only in this room, the chairs faced a huge wall of glass that opened onto something that resembled a low-budget living room.

We walked another couple of feet and stopped. The corridor ended at a large door. My escort grabbed the handle and looked to her left, into the command center. A buzzer sounded, and she pulled the door open, stepping aside so I could go through. It led into the living room space. Cheap couches, a television, and some wooden tables and chairs were scattered throughout a large, open area.

I hesitated, looking uncertainly at my guide. She smiled, inclining her head forward. "It's this way, Mr. Dylan."

Slowly, I walked into the crisis center. The woman, remaining in the hallway, shut the door behind me. I heard a clicking sound and knew that I was locked in. Several people sat in the command center, looking out into the living room. I felt suddenly anxious. It was as if they were watching an experiment, like, *Hey, throw him in there and let's see what happens!*

Glancing around, I saw that three people were sitting on the couches. One was alone, watching a baseball game on the television; the other two were huddled together and talking quietly. A few people were also sitting at one of the tables, conversing in low tones.

For a moment, I stood still, feeling exposed and on guard. A window opened into the command center from the living room. I walked over and peered inside. A woman, who I would later discover was a nurse, smiled across at me.

"Hello," she said. She glanced at several monitors next to her on the wall, which were clearly connected to video cameras throughout the facility. "Your wife is over there, Mr. Dylan," she said, pointing to several doors that I hadn't noticed. They were lined up on the right-hand side of the living area.

"Okay, thanks."

"No problem," she replied. "She's in the first bedroom."

I ambled slowly past the couches and peered inside the first room. I saw a couple of low mattresses on the floor, simple white sheets covering them. Mia was lying on one, staring up at the ceiling.

"Mia?" I asked, cautiously moving toward her. "Mia, it's me, how are you feeling?"

Mia turned her head in my direction. She didn't appear happy to see me. I wanted to rush over and kiss her, but given her expression, that didn't seem like a good idea. Instead, I moved to the foot of her mattress and took a seat. She didn't say anything.

Sitting on her bed, I could examine the rest of the room. The other mattress, identical to hers, was a couple of feet away. In addition to the beds, there were a closet and a few small bureaus. I immediately noticed the back of the bedroom door. It was covered with thousands of symbols, like mathematical calculations. It looked like someone had spent days doing advanced calculus on it with a black marker.

Mia continued to ignore me. We sat in silence for a few minutes.

"Is everything okay in here?" I finally asked.

"What do you think, Pat!" she barked at me. "Do you think it's okay in here?"

Things weren't starting off well.

"It looks okay." I glanced around the room. "I know that you've been seeing Dr. Martinez during the day."

"I can't believe you put me in here," she growled.

I already felt guilty for that, but what else could I have done? At least in here, with all of the video cameras and locked doors, she couldn't run away.

We sat quietly for another few minutes. Given her attitude, I was hesitant to initiate more conversation.

"I know what you're doing," she said, breaking the silence. "It's not going to work."

I had no idea what she was talking about; my pulse quickened. "Babe, what I am doing is trying to help you, that's all."

"You're helping me by locking me up in here?" Mia was sitting up now, facing me coldly, becoming more animated. "No, you can't fool me, Pat. I know what you're doing!"

My heart was beating rapidly now, and my palms were starting to sweat. I thought maybe I could change the subject, redirect her again. "Did you get the letters that we wrote to you?" I asked.

"Did you get the letters that we wrote to you?" she mimicked in a cruel voice, like you might expect hearing from the Joker in a Batman film. *"Did you get the letters?"*

I had another out-of-body experience. I was looking down on the scene, an impartial observer. My wife, the sweetest person I had ever known, had transformed. She was someone completely different, mean and confrontational.

"What's the matter, Pat? Upset because I know what's going on?!" she roared.

"I don't know what you are talking about," I implored. "The kids and I miss you, and we wanted to tell you how much we love you."

"Oh, c'mon, Pat. I can't believe you made the kids do that. You told them what to write," she sneered. "What did you have to give them to follow your orders? What did you bribe them with?"

We were the only two in the room, but I knew that the people in the command center had cameras hooked up. Maybe they were observing the interaction, or maybe it was just playing to an unwatched screen.

"What are you talking about?" I asked, as calmly as I could. "Why would I be bribing the kids?"

"Please, Pat, just stop. Stop with the games and tell me *the truth!*"

I gave an exasperated sigh. I couldn't believe that we were back to *the truth*. We were going in circles, getting nowhere.

"If you're not going to tell me the truth, then why don't you just leave?"

I stood up, backing away from her bed. "The truth, Mia? The truth is that I love you. The kids love you. We want you to get better and come home. That's the truth."

She rose and stomped over to stand an inch away from me, looking up insolently. "Oh, that's the truth, is it?" She turned and strode purposely over to the mattress. She grabbed something from behind it, between the bed and the wall, and wheeled around.

Taking a few steps toward me, she cocked her arm and flung it forward, throwing something violently in my direction. I flinched and braced for impact, but nothing hit me. Instead, the air exploded into what looked like confetti. A cloud of tiny pieces of paper fluttered into the air around us.

"There's your truth, Pat!" she yelled. "That's what I think of your truth!"

I looked at my chest and hands, suddenly realizing what she had thrown. Remnants of our homemade cards covered the floor, torn into a thousand bits. Several fragments had landed on me. Ripped pieces of our family picture were strewn everywhere.

She looked defiant and victorious, reveling in the shock apparent on my face. "That's right, Pat, I know what you're up to," she scoffed. "You can't fool me!"

"I'm not trying to fool you, Mia," I whispered. "I'm sorry that you think I am." I started backing out of the bedroom.

I was standing in the living room as she marched up to me again. "I want a divorce!" she shouted, and I imagined all the heads turning in our direction.

"Mia," I said calmly, not allowing myself to feel anything in the moment. "You don't know what you are talking about. You don't want a divorce, and neither do I. We love each other. We always have and we always will."

"Ha!" she cried, nearly spitting in my face. "I don't believe that anymore. I know what you're doing! Trying to steal the kids away from me. It won't work! I'm taking you down!"

I turned my head away, looking over to the command center window. The nurse was watching me attentively. I nodded to her, she gave a signal, and two huge guys, dressed identically, emerged from the far side of the room. I only meant for her to open the door so I could leave; but apparently, other protocols were in place.

Mia was still yelling, threatening me. "You think you can get better attorneys than I can? No way, Pat! I'm getting the best ones, and we are taking you down!"

The two guys grabbed Mia by either arm. She hadn't seen them coming and was startled. She started squirming, trying to escape their grasp. I could tell they were treating her as gently as they could, but it was still upsetting. She was screaming fiercely, "Let me go! LET ME GO!!"

I heard the buzzer sound, and the door opened. The same woman who had guided me in was standing in the corridor. I took one last look at the scuffle in front of me and then quickly walked out. As the door shut behind me, the two guards must have released Mia. She ran to it, her face against the window.

"COME BACK HERE, PAT!!" she shrieked. "I'M NOT DONE WITH YOU!!" She was furiously trying to open the door, fighting against the locked handle.

I followed closely behind my guide, turning as the hallway curved. Mia's shouting faded away; she must have given up when she couldn't see me anymore.

"Well, that was a good first visit," I said, feeling numb and trying to hold myself together.

The escort stopped at the entrance to the lobby, turning around with a gentle smile. "I'm sorry, Mr. Dylan," she said. "We see that kind of thing sometimes. Hopefully, tomorrow goes better."

"Not sure it could go much worse," I replied, slipping past her. As I collected my computer, both she and the receptionist drowned me with sympathetic looks. I escaped to the parking lot, dazed and crestfallen.

I will never forget that night, but neither will Mia ever remember it. Mental illness is bad enough; it interferes with rational thought, scrambles personalities. But before the psychotropic drugs start to help, they can exacerbate things. Poor Mia was on incredible amounts of mind-altering pharmaceuticals at the time.

Still, I was badly shaken. I didn't really think that she would want a divorce, but then again, I had no idea what was happening.

That night the scene replayed in my head hundreds of times, and I kept waking, staring into the blackness of our bedroom. I imagined the family photo as it had been, before Mia tore it apart. I wasn't going to let the illness destroy the life that we had built together. I kept repeating that promise to myself, like a call to arms.

I was tired the next morning, sitting at my desk and trying to concentrate, when my cell phone rang. "Hello, Mr. Dylan, this is Monica Perry," said a woman. "I'm a counselor at Pine Crest Middle School." My heart sank; it was Will again.

"Hello," I responded. "Are you calling about my son?"

"Yes, sir," she confirmed. "He is sitting here with me now."

"I see. May I speak with him?"

"Sure, hold on a second. I'll put him on."

"Dad?" I could tell that he had been crying.

"Will, what's wrong? Are you feeling the same as yesterday?"

"Yes." I waited for him to continue but heard silence.

"Remember when you got off the bus yesterday?" I asked. "You said you felt better after you went back to class. Do you think you can do that again today?"

"No. Dad, I just want to be with you. I want to come home."

"But Will, I'm not at home. I'm at my office," I said softly. "I need to work, and you need to go to school."

Silence.

"I know it's hard with Mom being sick, but she would want us to keep going. She'd want you to be in school."

A little muffled sniffling.

"We need to keep that in mind: What would Mom want us to do?"

"I know what Mom would want us to do," he admitted.

"Good. Look, do me a favor. Give it your best shot. Stay there with your counselor for a little bit, until you are composed, and then go back to class. I'll be here at work, thinking of you. Give class an hour. That's all I'm asking. And then, if you still can't handle it, I'll come and get you."

"Okay, Dad. I'll try."

"That's all I can ask, Will. Just give it a shot. I love you."

"I love you, too, Dad."

"Mr. Dylan?" The counselor was back on the line.

"Yes, hi," I said, trying to sound confident. "I know Will is having a hard time, and I wanted to explain."

"Please do. He was down here yesterday, too." She didn't sound mad, only concerned.

"We are going through a health crisis in our family right now. My wife is very sick. She was in the emergency room, and now she's back in the hospital," I explained, conveniently leaving out the mental health part.

"I'm so sorry to hear that, Mr. Dylan."

"Yeah, it hasn't been easy," I said. "We're doing the best we can. She's going to get better, but Will, he's worried about his mom."

"Okay, well, we'll keep an eye on him," she replied, and I could tell that she was smiling down at him when she said it. "I hope that your wife recovers quickly."

Hanging up, I exhaled deeply, acknowledging once again the serious ramifications that Mia's illness could have on the kids. I was still thinking about this when I drove to the crisis center for daytime visiting hours. Once at the GTC, however, my thoughts immediately shifted to Mia. Would she be in attack mode again?

To my surprise, my visit was immediately accepted. This time, the person who came out to greet me was the same young woman who had admitted Mia. She had a kind disposition, dark hair, and a tattoo on her arm.

"Mr. Dylan," she said, ushering me into the hallway, "my name is Autumn. I work with Dr. Martinez and have been spending a lot of time with Mia."

"Nice to meet you," I responded. "You're lucky you weren't with her last night. She wasn't in a very good mood."

"Yeah, I heard about that. Mia does go through phases. I think you'll find her much easier to deal with today."

She opened the door to the crisis center, stepping aside as I walked in. Mia was slumped on one of the couches, staring indifferently ahead. I walked over slowly, sitting down next to her.

"Hi, Mia," I said with uncertainty.

She glanced at me. "Hi." She was heavily sedated, her voice groggy.

"How are you doing?" I sensed that she was too subdued to start berating me.

"I'm okay," she said in a sleepy voice, glancing around the room. "Look at this place, though; it's messed up. I think there are drug deals going on in the back." She motioned with her head toward the corner of the room, but no one was there. "And the people tell me fake names. One girl wants me to call her Autumn. She'll probably start going by Winter next week."

I wasn't sure how to respond as Mia's slow drawl continued. "They poison the water in the drinking fountain here, too. Stay away from that."

I decided to change the subject. "You look tired, babe."

"I had to clean the door all morning."

"Clean the door?"

"Yeah, I wrote on it. It was important, but they made me erase it."

Of course, I thought to myself. *All of those mathematical calculations scribbled on the back of the bedroom door were hers.*

The whole visit went that way. We mostly sat in silence; Mia was a zombie, spaced out and tired. The long gaps in conversation were frustrating.

After visiting hours, I returned home feeling dejected. My parents were out, so I wandered into the bedroom and collapsed onto the bed. I knew staying upbeat was important, especially for the kids, but I couldn't shake the feeling of hopelessness.

I was thinking about what life would be like after my parents left. I didn't know how I was going to juggle everything. I was spending half of my time at the treatment center. Mia's condition was swinging wildly from belligerent to apathetic, and that was when she actually agreed to see me. Will was balancing on the edge of his own emotional breakdown. Jamie was carrying on as if nothing were wrong, and that didn't seem right, either. I hadn't had to worry about meals or laundry over the past two weeks, but that was going to change. And then there was work. Although my employers were supportive, I was only putting in a couple of hours a day.

The kids were depending on me. Mia was counting on me, too, not the drugged-up person sitting in the crisis center, but the compassionate woman with whom I had fallen in love. I couldn't let her down. But how long would it take for her to get better?

I closed my eyes, tears starting to form. What was even wrong with her? Would we ever figure it out?

Sprawled on the bed, consumed by these questions, I suddenly heard someone knocking. My parents wouldn't have knocked. Puzzled, I stood and tried to compose myself as our dog's barking echoed through the house. Walking to the front door, I pulled it open, ready to sign for a delivery or greet the neighbor. Instead, I froze in surprise.

There, standing on the porch, was someone completely unexpected. He had left the country a dozen years before, and I hadn't seen him since. Truth be told, I wasn't sure that I would ever see him again.

I couldn't believe my eyes. He looked different: older and thinner, with a darker tan and longer hair. But his sharp blue eyes still carried a look of mischief.

It was Mia's younger brother, Luke.

10.

THE LOST CUBAN

Ringside
"Miss You"
2:19–2:48

Although I met Mia's parents briefly at graduation, the full personality of her family didn't come through until I traveled down to Florida. I grew up in a small town in Indiana and, other than a trip to Mexico, had never left the country. Being in Miami was like being in another world.

But one thing was familiar: Mia's family felt just like mine. Cousins, aunts, uncles, and grandparents all gathered for the holidays. They were loud and passionate. It was as if my relatives had been taught Spanish and transported to the tropics.

That was the first time I met Mark. He and Mia were similar, both studious and meticulous. They took after Marcos, who was an engineer. In fact, they both resembled him, with their brown eyes and more aquiline noses. Celia and Luke, with their blue eyes and outgoing personalities, were more like Lucia's side of the family. They were both smart, too; all the siblings had graduated from

Georgetown. But Celia and Luke were less inclined to study, and they didn't like to follow rules—especially Luke.

He greeted me with enthusiasm every time I saw him. "Patricio, I got nothing but love for you, brother!" He would come in with the bro handshake and then pull me into a hug.

Mia's extended family was close, but her immediate family was even closer. That being said, I always sensed that the strict upbringing had left some lingering resentment. Mark and Mia had buckled down and obeyed, but Celia and Luke had rebelled.

It still came as a shock when Luke disappeared. Well, I guess he didn't really disappear; he told everyone he was leaving. One morning, he got into his car and started driving. He drove straight through Mexico and half of Central America and didn't stop until he reached Costa Rica.

Shortly after, Mark went searching to make sure his little brother was alright. He found Luke living in a beachside shack with no running water, working as the crocodile man on some backwoods-type jungle adventure. The photo Mark brought back still hangs on his parents' wall: Luke using a dead chicken to lure a twelve-foot reptile out of a dirty lagoon.

After that, we heard snippets about Luke once or twice a year. He would call home on Mother's Day, or he'd send an email for Christmas. There was no pattern to his updates. Every time, he was living in a new place: Mexico, Brazil, Italy, Thailand, Japan, Tunisia, Siberia, the Philippines, Puerto Rico. He never stayed in one place long.

All kinds of theories were proposed to explain why Luke had fled. He had racked up loads of credit card debt, and the banks were after him. He was on the mob's hit list for some unnamed transgression. They all seemed far-fetched to me. I assumed that he just didn't want to live the American, material-driven lifestyle.

Whatever the reason, the family was never whole after Luke left. Marcos and Lucia included him at the end of every grace. *And God willing, please watch over Luke and keep him safe, wherever he is.* Seven grandkids had been born, and none of them had met their long-lost uncle. I had only known Luke for a short while, and I missed him. Mia longed desperately to see him again. Most of us doubted that he would ever come back.

And then, on that otherwise hopeless day in October, I opened the door and found him standing on our doorstep.

***

"Patricio," he greeted me, but not with his usual excitement. He was more restrained. "I heard about Mia. I'm here for you."

Luke was like the magical character from a fairy tale, appearing when you needed him most. I shook my head. I couldn't believe he was actually standing in front of me.

He smiled. "Yo, I still got nothing but love for you, brother." He didn't even go for the usual handshake; he just came forward with a hug.

"Luke, wow, it's so great to see you!" I exclaimed after his presence finally settled in. I went to grab his luggage, but all he had was a green rucksack thrown across his shoulder and a long, thin canvas bag leaning against the wall next to him. He noticed me eyeing the bag warily; it had the shape of a shotgun.

"*Mira*," he said. Luke had a habit of throwing Spanish words into any conversation. "These are my spearguns. I thought I could do some spearfishing while I'm here, yeah?"

Luke was in his late thirties, but he looked younger than his age. His long dark hair was pulled tightly into a ponytail, the brown hue matching that of his short-cropped goatee. Their Cuban heritage meant that Mia and her siblings tanned quickly whenever they spent time in the sun. Luke lived on the beach and in the water; his skin was a dark bronze.

He didn't have an ounce of fat, a natural consequence of living off the sea. But neither was he skinny. His legs and arms were sinewy, the result of fending for himself in God knows what kind of exploits. He was good-looking, and I had no doubt that women in far-off places found his swashbuckling persona attractive. His piercing blue eyes always seemed to be laughing at the world and its inability to control him.

He was wearing a worn-out tank top and a pair of loose-fitting board shorts, both of which had seen way too much mileage. His flip-flops were superfluous; he spent most of his life barefoot. I was pretty sure that all of his worldly belongings were in that rucksack. He didn't care for material goods; the spearguns and an underwater camera were his prized possessions.

"Um, okay," I said, glancing uncomfortably at the canvas bag, "but can you put them up on the shelf in the garage? I don't like the idea of having spearguns in the house."

"Aces." He grinned.

We walked into the kitchen. "Where have you been living?" I asked. "Last I heard you were in Italy, maybe, or Thailand?"

"Yeah," he smirked, "that was a while ago. I been living in Roatán."

"Roatán? Where the hell is that?"

"It's an island off the coast of Honduras, near the second-largest barrier reef in the world. I been working as a dive instructor there for four, maybe five months now."

"Man, you must be in heaven then." But I wondered how he had ended up at our house. "Luke, how did you know? And how did you get here?"

"Yo, I got an email from Celia a few days ago sayin' some shit about Mia. It sounded bad, man. Celia be tripping. So, I packed up my stuff, found a flight . . . *pa pa pa, pe pe pe* . . . borrowed a car from my parents."

For the record, I wasn't sure if *pa pa pa, pe pe pe* was a colloquial expression that Luke picked up somewhere or a phrase he had created. But he used it all the time. It basically meant the same as "et cetera" or "I'm skipping a bunch of stuff, so try to keep up."

He was looking around the house, his eyes moving out to our lanai and the pool. He paused. "Damn, dude, y'all been working hard, yeah?"

"Oh, sorry, I forgot that you've never been here," I said, laughing. "Thanks, we like it. Can I show you around?"

"Nah," he responded, suddenly serious again. "Tell me, what's going on with Mia?"

I gave him a short update, but he had already heard most of it from Celia and Mark. But even they didn't know what had happened recently at the crisis center, with the torn-up letters and scrawled-out bedroom door.

"Dude, that's some fucked-up shit," he said.

"Yeah, it is," I agreed, "but Mia isn't thinking straight. It's not like she's meaning to act this way."

"Nuh-uh, I get you," he responded with a look of understanding.

"But Luke, it can be tough. Celia had a difficult time with it."

"Bro, I got stories for you. I seen some shit in my day. It ain't nothing I can't handle."

I could only imagine the things that Luke had experienced. I smiled and shook my head. "I'm sure that's true. How long can you stick around?"

"Long as it takes, *hermano*, long as it takes. I got no commitments or deadlines."

"Wow," I said, relieved. "I can't tell you how much that means, for you to put your life on hold for us."

"It's family, Patricio."

Luke said it with finality, like nothing else mattered. Mia had always told me that he was the most caring of her siblings. She would go on and on about how much attention he paid to their grandmother or how he treated their mom. In that moment, I finally understood what she meant.

"Thank you," I said, holding his gaze. A moment passed, and then I remembered. "Oh, Luke, my parents will be in the guest room for one more night. But we can put you on the futon in the study until tomorrow."

"No, man, I don't do beds. Not my thing."

"What?" I asked, wondering if I understood him correctly. "Did you say that you don't sleep on beds?"

"*Sí*," he confirmed. "Beds make you soft. So long as you got a floor, I'll be good."

Having him around was going to be an adventure. "Okay," I laughed, "we've got plenty of floors. Take your pick!"

He threw his rucksack in our back room and was off again. He planned to find a dive shop and sharpen his spearguns. Watching him leave, I realized how perfect he would be for the situation. Mia would enjoy spending time with him, and Luke could certainly handle her condition. He could stay with her during the day and then camp in the back of our house at night. And the kids? They would absolutely love him.

When they came home, I informed them of Luke's arrival. Jamie didn't know what to think; she only knew her Uncle Luke from stories. As for Will, he was in a great mood when he got off the bus. Hearing about Luke only widened the smile on his face.

"Dad, I went back to class, just like you said, and after a while I felt better," he said. "Once it was lunchtime, I knew I could make it!"

"That's great, Will! See, if you stay in class, there's nothing to worry about."

"Yeah, I just wish I could tell myself that in the mornings." Will could talk rationally about his feelings at home. "It's weird, Dad. It's like I get worried that I'm going to start getting worried. Does that make any sense?"

"It's hard for me to understand, but it does make sense. Anxiety runs in our family." He was listening attentively. "Mom has always been a worrier, and so has Uncle Brad. They'd probably get it, but I've never had to deal with anything like that."

"It's really hard when it starts happening."

"Isn't there anything you can do to calm yourself down?"

"I try, but it's like my thoughts get out of control."

"That sounds scary," I admitted. "Hey, Will, what if I found someone you could talk to about it, a person trained in dealing with anxiety? Would you be open to that?"

"Sure, I guess, if you think it might help."

I added one more thing to my list, putting it at the top. Maybe Dr. Martinez would have a recommendation, or perhaps the school counselor? Either way, I had to identify a good therapist for Will.

Dinner that night was a riot. Luke returned from his errands, and everyone was excited to see him. The kids were captivated. We had read *Treasure Island* more than once, and they viewed their uncle as some kind of modern-day pirate.

When I arrived at the crisis center Friday night, I was hopeful that Mia would have more energy than earlier in the day. However, the visit was basically a repeat of the last session. She sat disengaged and half-comatose, and I tried to remain as patient as possible. I left with a familiar feeling of remorse.

The next morning began with much anticipation. My parents were leaving, but before they did, we were all headed to the British restaurant for Jamie's makeup tea party. We tried to convince Luke to join us, but he wanted to check out the local fishing scene.

I was in a good mood driving from the tea shop to the GTC, and it only improved once I saw Mia. She was sitting at one of the wooden tables, appearing awake and normal. Our conversation was better, too. She asked about the kids, wanting to know how they were doing. It was almost as if the psychosis had cleared completely. Indeed, all seemed fine until visiting hours were over.

"Take me with you, Pat," she pleaded. "I don't want to stay here anymore. I miss home."

She was talking so rationally, and the way she was beseeching me, it broke my heart to answer. "Babe, I wish I could, but I can't. You need to stay here until the doctors release you."

"But I miss you, and I miss the kids."

"We miss you, too," I said, standing and giving her a hug. "You'll be home with us soon." I said it with conviction, and I believed it. She seemed so much better.

"No!" Mia demanded, her voice rising. "I'm coming home with you right now!"

"But you can't," I reiterated in a calm voice, hoping to soothe her. "I'll be back tonight."

"Tonight isn't good enough!" she yelled. "I want to leave now!" She was blocking my way, looking defiant again.

"Mia, please, I'll see you soon."

"No!" she cried for the second time, an angry glare in her eyes. "Get me out of here, Pat! Get me out!"

"I told you, babe, I can't do that," I implored as my fight-or-flight response started to fire. "I wish that I could."

"It's not fair that you get to go!" Mia screamed, following me across the room. "I'M LEAVING WITH YOU!!"

Then many things happened at once. The two large workers materialized out of nowhere. They each grabbed ahold of Mia. At the same time, the person who had escorted me that afternoon emerged at the door. "Mr. Dylan, visiting hours are over."

"I know," I answered, glancing behind me, "but I'd like to make sure that Mia is okay."

She was fighting against the men who held her. They probably outweighed Mia by a hundred pounds each, but they were struggling to maintain control. She was kicking her legs and wrenching her arms, shrieking, "GET OFF ME!! I'LL CALL THE POLICE!!"

My instincts told me to protect my wife by ripping her from the arms of her captors. But Mia didn't look like someone who needed rescuing. She looked more like a wild animal, with vicious eyes and a savage face.

"Mr. Dylan?" The escort had come to my side. "Please come with me. Now."

But I was mesmerized, held in place, adrenaline pumping. I was just about to jump into the fray when a hand clutched my elbow.

"Mr. Dylan, please," begged the woman, pulling my arm. "We've seen this before. It will be best for your wife if you leave."

Her voice broke me out of a trance. Maybe she was right; they were trained professionals. Without losing sight of Mia, I backed my way into the corridor. I watched through the window as the combat intensified. The two guards had grappled Mia to the ground.

"What are they doing to her!" I cried.

"They are giving her a shot to calm her down," explained my escort. "It happens, Mr. Dylan." My guide kept nudging me until she had led me down the hall and into the lobby.

"Trust me," she said as we emerged into the waiting room, "Mia will be fine. Sometimes people fight to get out, but they aren't ready yet. The doctors will determine when it is appropriate for your wife to leave."

"Yeah, okay," I responded gloomily. It was discouraging to move so quickly from hope to despair.

The drive home was miserable. I stopped by a Cuban cafeteria on the way and picked up black beans, rice, shredded pork, and plantains. I knew Luke would enjoy it, and the food would remind the kids of Mia.

Saturday night's dinner went a long way toward cheering me up. It was the first time the kids and I shared a meal alone with Luke. Will and Jamie began what would become a favorite pastime: asking their uncle extreme questions about his life.

"Uncle Luke, what's the most dangerous animal you've ever been up close to?" Jamie wanted to know.

"Most dangerous animal?" Luke repeated, amused and thinking carefully. "I'd want to say tiger sharks, yeah? One time, I was diving off Thailand and this monster fifteen-foot *tiburón tigre* came out of nowhere." Will and Jamie were immediately enthralled.

"His eyes were spooky, too," Luke continued. "I'm not even kidding you, either. Mira, he was looking right at me." Luke split his fingers apart and pointed them to his eyes. "Like he was watching me!"

The kids sat spellbound as Luke paused dramatically. Then suddenly, he sat back and resumed eating. "But yo, that's probably not the most dangerous. Everyone thinks sharks are dangerous, but they ain't too bad. I'll tell you what is, though—hippos."

The three of us looked at each other and smirked, assuming that he was joking. "Hippos?" I asked. "Where did you see those?"

"Africa," answered Luke, his eyes reengaging us. He was deadly serious again. "And I'll tell you what, them bitches is scary, bro. Unpredictable." I gave him a look like, *C'mon, man, watch the language.* He nodded and continued.

"With a hippo, you don't know they're there, see? One minute you be on your raft or whatnot, all at peace and such . . . *pa pa pa, pe pe pe* . . . and then wham! Them hippos attack. And they got huge teeth, see, I'm talking over a foot long!" He made a motion with his hands, showing us how big the incisors of a hippopotamus could be. He had the kids hooked again. This went on for the rest of the meal.

As I drove to evening visiting hours, I realized just how uplifting Luke's presence would be. Not only did he have an endless number of outlandish stories, but he had found a favorite audience in the kids. When I neared the treatment center, however, I became nervous, wondering if Mia would put up another fight.

I found her highly sedated, probably the result of whatever they had given her when I left. In fact, she was so tired that she went to bed early. It was strange, tucking her into the mattress on the floor. But it made me feel good, like I was bringing her some comfort. She was asleep before I left.

Back home, I finally dealt with dozens of unanswered voice mails that were plaguing my phone. Most were about Mia, many from friends who were concerned because she had stopped responding to them.

About halfway through the messages, I heard the voice of one of the doctors from Mia's former practice. "Pat, our office has been receiving calls from Mia. She says she's locked up at the Gulfshore Treatment Center and needs our help. Is everything okay?" I looked at the date; it was several days old. "Can you please call me?" the doctor finished. "We're all very worried about her."

But Celia took Mia's cell phone when she was admitted to the crisis center! I thought frantically. *How is she making calls?*

Flustered, I immediately dialed the doctor. She was one of Mia's closest work colleagues and answered quickly. I confessed that Mia was suffering from serious anxiety and that her psychiatrist believed the treatment center was the best place for her. I didn't mention psychosis, and the doctor didn't question me further, but she was an expert. She must have known that the situation was far more serious.

Checking in with the receptionist the next day, I asked, "Do you know how someone here could have gained access to a phone?"

"Why, yes, Mr. Dylan, there is a phone for our patients to use," the receptionist replied, as if nothing could be more normal. But her response startled me. Trying to keep Mia's illness a secret was a losing battle if she had access to a phone.

As discouraged as I was, seeing Mia made me feel better. Her thought process was even clearer than the prior afternoon. Her personality remained flat and unemotional, but she wasn't warning me about lurking dangers. And she wasn't nearly as groggy as the night before.

As our time together drew to a close, I finally mustered the courage to broach the question. "Mia, have you been calling anyone while you've been in here?"

"I think I might have called my work a few times," she said, "but that's the only number I could remember."

It was encouraging; contacting her work was unfortunate, but at least the damage had been limited. I was concerned about leaving, but Mia escorted me to the door without protest. Surprisingly, I left the GTC feeling upbeat for the first time.

More good news arrived later that afternoon. Dr. Martinez called and said that, in his opinion, Mia's condition was no longer an emergency. He believed that the Seroquel had finally addressed her psychosis and that she could come home the following day. But she wasn't fully recovered, and for that reason he wanted to see me before discharging her. We agreed to meet at the crisis center the following morning.

I was excited to welcome Mia back, but the kids seemed apprehensive. She had been acting strange before going to the treatment center, and that was after they had already been told that she was better. Luke seemed pleased when I told him, but we hadn't yet discussed a plan for managing things once she returned.

"I'm assuming you can watch Mia during the day, when I'm at work, and provide updates periodically?" I asked.

"That sounds like a plan," he said. "I been thinking, though. I don't have a phone. Maybe we use email to communicate, or Skype?"

It hadn't occurred to me. Of course Luke didn't have a cell phone; he slept on the floor of a dive shop on a remote island.

"Hmm, that's a problem. Okay, what's your Skype handle?"

"*Cubano Perdido*," he answered, smirking.

I shook my head. "Lost Cuban" was certainly the handle most befitting Luke. However, given that only one computer was available to him in our study, and that he might need to contact me quickly, Luke agreed to buy a cheap mobile phone. I offered to pay, but he wouldn't hear of it.

My visit with Mia on Sunday night was similar to the one during the day. I expected that now that the psychosis had cleared, her personality would start to resurface, but I was wrong. Her thoughts were coherent, but she was apathetic and listless.

When I was tucking Will into bed later that night, I could sense his nervousness about returning to school after the weekend. He was even worse the next morning. I tried to calm him down the best I could before sending him off, but he was half-paralyzed with anxiety. When I saw his call an hour later, I wasn't surprised.

"Sorry, Dad," he whimpered. "I tried . . . I really did."

"I'm sure you did," I reassured him.

"I just wanted to hear your voice. I just wanted to make sure you were there."

"I'm always here, Will."

"I know," he sniffed, "I know."

"Now, see if you can go back to class. It's only until lunchtime."

"Okay, I know."

"Love you, Will. Please let me talk to your counselor."

"I love you, too, Dad. Okay."

As soon as I heard Will transfer the phone, I wasted no time in questioning Mrs. Perry. "Good morning," I said. "I was wondering if you knew anyone who might be able to work with Will, maybe give him some tools for managing his anxiety?"

"Why yes, Mr. Dylan," she said, "I could give you several names, but I think the best would be Matthew Brown. He has worked with several of the kids I advise, and people have really good things to say about him."

"Matthew Brown?" I confirmed. "I'll call him."

A couple of hours later, Autumn was ushering me through the corridor of the crisis center. I didn't realize that offices were located on the right-hand side of the hallway. Autumn opened a door, and I saw Dr. Martinez sitting at a desk. He stood and greeted me.

"Pat, as you know, Mia is on a high dose of Seroquel," he began after I had taken a seat. "And she needs to stay at that level for a while."

"Okay, that shouldn't be a problem."

"Well, it might be. These drugs can be difficult. First, they make you tired. But it's more than that, they make you feel sort of dulled, like you aren't really yourself."

"Ah, right." I nodded my head. "I've noticed that about Mia."

"I'm sure you have. And also, the medication can make people gain weight. It slows the metabolism and makes people hungry. It's a double whammy."

"Alright, but these symptoms aren't long term, are they?"

"They will dissipate if Mia stops taking the Seroquel, yes."

"And when will that be?"

"Well, that depends. It's not our job, here at the crisis center, to make a full diagnosis. We do our best in the time that we have, but Mia should be seeing someone regularly."

"Yes, well, I expect that she'll continue seeing you."

He smiled. "I appreciate that, Pat, but I should tell you that people often switch psychiatrists after coming to the crisis center. Being with me reminds them too much of their time here. If that happens with Mia, I won't be offended."

"Really? Okay, well, I guess we'll see. But right now, you've spent the most time with her. What do you think is going on?"

He thought carefully before answering. "It's a strange case. The original diagnosis of brief reactive psychosis might be correct. But I think it must be related to bipolar disorder. She seemed manic when I first saw her, and that didn't change when she was admitted here. Mania can frequently turn psychotic. I see it all the time."

"I've been reading about bipolar, though, and you were right. It's not bipolar without depression."

"Yes, that's what makes it strange." He sat in thought again before snapping back to the task at hand. "I don't have a good answer for you. But now, it's time to get Mia home."

Soon, Mia and I were walking out of the lobby. I had her duffel bag in hand, and it felt strangely like she had been released from prison. I thought she would be happy, but her personality was as blunted as it had been the day before.

"There's a surprise waiting at home," I said as we started the drive. "Someone came into town to spend time with you, someone you haven't seen in a long time." I thought hearing about Luke would brighten her mood.

"What are you talking about?" She sounded frustrated.

"Luke. He's at our house! He came to see you."

She looked confused. "Luke? Why would Luke be at our house?"

"He came home because he heard you were having a difficult time, and he wanted to help." I expected some sign of excitement, but she only frowned.

With the benefit of hindsight, I understand Mia's reaction. After spending a week in a mental health facility, she was thinking more clearly, or so she had been told, but she didn't remember much. And then abruptly, I told her that Luke was in town, someone whom she hadn't seen for over a decade. That wasn't normal, and it made her nervous. Was her mind fooling her? Was I trying to fool her?

Of course, at the time I didn't realize this. So I tried again to cheer her up. "Anyway, the kids will be excited to see you when we get home."

"Pat, why would the kids be home?" she asked, becoming angrier. "The kids are in school right now."

"I pulled them out early so we could spend time together. Luke is picking them up. They should be home when we get there."

"Whatever, Pat, whatever." She shook her head in disgust and ignored me the rest of the trip.

Her reaction was equally chilly when the kids greeted her in the kitchen. She hugged them, but she didn't show any interest. This was also true when she saw Luke. Lunch was awkward, much like our meals before Mia went to the crisis center. It didn't faze Luke, but the kids and I were disappointed.

After lunch, Luke took the opportunity to go fishing. I suggested that the rest of us play board games, something we had always enjoyed doing together in the past. But the feeling of discomfort permeated the afternoon. Mia left abruptly after an hour, saying she was tired, and the kids retreated to their bedrooms.

I remained sitting among the games. Having Mia around wasn't going to improve our situation. Her sour disposition made everyone uneasy, and the fact that her personality was so different was distressing. Hopefully, she would start to act more like herself soon, but I didn't know if that was possible while she was on so much medication.

I decided to check on Will. He was at his desk, doing homework. "How was the rest of your day, kid?" I asked.

"It was okay." He sounded dispirited. "I don't know what happens to me at school, but I'm really not looking forward to tomorrow morning."

Sensing that he wanted to be alone, my thoughts moved to Jamie. When I walked into her room, she was lying down on the bed, reading. "Can I talk to you for a sec?"

Jamie put her book down and sat up. "What is it, Daddy?"

Closing the door, I paced across the room to the end of her bed. "I've been meeting with Will. Given everything that's going on with Mommy, he's been worrying a lot." She was focused on me, her young eyes looking intently into mine. She didn't say anything. "And, well, I thought maybe you'd want to talk about it, too."

"Talk about what?"

"Talk about how you're feeling. You know, with every-thing that's going on with Mommy."

"Oh, I know what's going on with Mommy."

"You do?"

"Yes, I know exactly what's going on."

"Really? What?" I was surprised, but maybe she had been reading about mental health. She was a precocious child.

"Mommy was taken by aliens," Jamie said, her voice solemn. "They have her up on their spaceship. And then they put a robot in her place, hoping we wouldn't notice."

I wasn't sure how to respond. "Jamie, sweetie, you don't really believe that, do you?"

"Do you?" she retorted.

"No, I don't think that. I think Mommy has an illness and needs our help."

"Okay." She grabbed her book. "Is that it, Daddy?"

I wanted to keep talking. I was pretty sure she was joking, but I wasn't certain. However, Jamie clearly wanted to lie back down and continue reading.

"Uh, yeah, I guess so," I mumbled, leaning over to hug her.

By the time I reached the door, she was already engrossed in her book again. I walked out, adding another priority to my list: Jamie definitely needed to see a professional, too.

11.

THE STRANGER

Bill Withers
"Ain't No Sunshine"
1:14–1:35

Mia and I got engaged two years after graduation. I planned an elaborate setup for asking her, and Mia acted surprised, but that was only to humor me. By then, she knew the question was coming.

For Mia and her parents, it was important that we marry in the Catholic Church. To do so, we had to attend something called "Pre-Cana Weekend." Essentially, it consisted of a two-day conversation about our relationship. During the day, we either sat around listening to couples talk about the challenges of marriage, or we were split into groups and asked to examine various topics.

The lectures could be long and disheartening. One couple spent an hour telling us how difficult marriage could be: "You have to be willing to wake up every morning and see the same person lying next to you," the husband remarked. "You have to be ready to live with that."

"Yes," the wife added, "and sometimes you'll start to question your decision."

I knew that getting married meant seeing the same person next to me every day. That was the whole point. I couldn't think of anything better, and I didn't expect that to ever change. Still, they kept droning on and on: "You might find that you want a change, but in the Catholic Church, marriage is a sacrament. It can't be changed."

I looked around the room like, *Don't these people already know this? Did all of these other couples decide to get married without knowing what they were signing up for?*

Apparently, the answer to that question was yes, which became clear in the group exercises when they asked us about specific issues. For example, the leader would say something like, "I'd like everyone to take out a piece of paper. Now, without sharing it, please write down if you want to have children, and, if the answer is yes, write down how many you'd like to have."

After recording our responses, we would exchange papers with our partners and compare. For Mia and me, this was all review; we had discussed every topic before. However, some of the participants discovered that they had opposite answers. For one couple next to us, the question about kids probably broke up their engagement. Mia and I were dumbstruck. How could they have agreed to marriage without knowing the answers to these essential questions?

Pre-Cana might have been necessary for some people, but it wasn't for us. We both believed that trust and honesty were vital to any relationship. We both wanted children, somewhere between two and three if we could. And yes, even though I was Protestant, we both agreed that raising our kids Catholic was important.

Other topics were discussed, one applicable to this story. We were asked what we would do if our spouse became sick, if they got cancer, if they became paralyzed. For Mia and me, this was easy: you stick by your spouse. That's what best friends do. That's what people who love each other do.

They didn't ask us, at Pre-Cana, what we would do if our spouse became mentally ill and their personality and character completely changed. Nor had Mia and I ever discussed it.

I would have to figure that answer out on my own.

***

After she was released from the crisis center, Mia was distant and ill-tempered. She always seemed on the brink of exploding, and it kept the rest of us on edge.

I could sense that the kids were having a hard time understanding their mom's dark personality. A few days after her return, I broached the subject. They were both doing homework at the kitchen table while I prepared dinner. Mia, who was spending most of her time in the bedroom, wasn't around.

"You've probably noticed that Mom hasn't been acting like herself even though she's out of the hospital," I said, watching for their reaction.

Jamie didn't look up; she probably didn't feel like talking about space robots again. Will's eyes didn't leave his notebook, either, but he responded quietly, "She's never happy anymore. She's always angry."

"I know, it's because of her medication. The doctors have given her medicine to help her brain heal. And it's working, but unfortunately, it makes her really grumpy."

Our kids were good students, but they had never been so absorbed in their studies.

"But it's only for a while. The medicine will help her get better, and then she'll be back to her usual self. I promise." Even as I said it, I knew that my empty assurances were losing credibility. The kids didn't respond, and my talk didn't help them reconcile what was happening. Will continued to struggle in school, and Jamie remained an enigma.

Luke was great. He understood the effects that the drugs were having and wasn't bothered by Mia's behavior. I didn't get the sense that they were spending quality time together. It was more like he was a prison guard, making sure that she didn't leave the house.

As for my relationship with Mia, it couldn't have been much worse. Although she had withdrawn from everyone, she was most resentful toward me. She wouldn't forgive me for sending her to the crisis center. She asserted that the GTC had been a traumatizing experience. I didn't doubt that it was upsetting, but some of what she said was hard to believe.

For example, Mia claimed that she had been raped. Clearly, this was a serious charge, and I didn't take it lightly. But every square inch of that place was monitored by cameras. Surely, a rape couldn't have gone unnoticed, especially with all of the nurses and guards standing by to de-escalate a situation. Plus, I had trust in Dr. Martinez and the other GTC workers with whom I had interacted. It was the word of a respected institution and trusted caregivers against a highly medicated, mentally ill patient.

Still, Mia demanded that representatives from the treatment center answer for their supposed crimes. She issued a complaint, and a meeting was promptly arranged. I wanted to support my wife, but her assertion seemed almost impossible.

I didn't have much time to dwell on it, however; the next two weeks were filled with appointments. We had a follow-up meeting scheduled with Dr. Martinez, and we also had other checkups that Mia had planned months in advance.

The meeting with Dr. Martinez was short, given that we had seen him so recently. He reiterated his belief that Mia's illness was somehow related to bipolar disorder and instructed her to continue the high dosage of Seroquel for the foreseeable future. He was trying to speak with her directly, but she kept ignoring him.

"There's no way I am seeing that guy again," she declared once we were back in the car. "I don't trust him."

Even though Dr. Martinez had warned me about the possibility, it was hard to believe. "I like him," I said. "He's smart and understanding, and he's been so supportive."

Mia didn't respond, so I added, "He has really been there for us."

"Been there for us, Pat!" she spat. "Us? He might have been there for you, but he has not been there for me! He kept me locked up in that place. No, Pat, that's it. Find someone else."

I resigned myself to identifying a new psychiatrist. My strategy was to filter online reviews based on ratings and availability. After several hours of research and phone calls, I presented three names to Mia. She randomly selected Dr. Eduardo Rojas and told me to schedule a meeting with him.

The next day, I drove her to an appointment with her gynecologist. Mia wasn't psychotic anymore. When people interacted with her, the things she said made sense. She remained paranoid, but it wasn't obvious. She saved her exaggerated suspicions for me, not sharing them with others.

Although I had never met Dr. Leonetti, Mia had been seeing her for years. When we were called from the waiting room, a nurse took Mia's weight and blood pressure. "So, Mia," she asked, sitting at a computer, "are you taking any new medications?"

Mia scowled at me, making it clear that I should answer, so I rattled off the various drugs and dosages. After flashing a startled expression, the nurse started typing furiously. She then escorted us to an examining room and asked us to wait.

Dr. Leonetti came in about twenty minutes later with an air of concern. She was accompanied by the same nurse.

"Tell me, Mia," the doctor began, "how have you been doing?"

"Not so well," admitted Mia. "I've had a lot of anxiety lately and am on medication for it."

"Right." Dr. Leonetti looked over at her computer screen. "Everything okay now?"

"I feel better now, yes. Thank you."

"That's good," the doctor said, still studying her monitor. "Is this your husband?"

"Yes, it is," replied Mia. I stood to introduce myself.

The doctor then began her gynecological review. She asked several basic questions, typing in the responses.

"Alright," she said, glancing through her notes, "looks like we are due for a mammogram after the general exam. Do you have any other concerns I should know about?"

"Yes. I'd like a full test for sexually transmitted diseases, including HIV."

This last comment caught my attention.

"Okay, we can do that," replied Dr. Leonetti. It appeared that she didn't find this request out of the ordinary, but I sure did. It added weight to Mia's claim that she had been raped. Why else would she want to run all of those tests? The doctor must have been wondering the same thing.

"Tell me, Mia, do you have reason to believe that you might have contracted an STD?" she asked.

Mia was looking at Dr. Leonetti. Then, deliberately, she turned my way, narrowing her eyes in an accusatory fashion. "I have my reasons," she said menacingly, glaring at me, before swiveling her head back toward the doctor.

"I see," said Dr. Leonetti with an uncomfortable pause. "Okay, we'll plan to run a complete battery of STD tests for you."

I could only imagine what the doctor and nurse were thinking. I didn't know if Mia truly had a concern or if she only wanted to embarrass me. I sank lower into my chair for the remainder of the appointment.

Mia never apologized for insinuating that I was cheating on her; in fact, she never mentioned it again. We weren't talking much. She remained standoffish and irritable, and spent most of her time alone. It was futile trying to engage her in conversation; every exchange ended in disagreement, or she would stop talking abruptly, completely ignoring everything that was said. I learned to avoid her, and the kids did, too. She was living in our house, but she was a stranger.

As upsetting as the experience with Dr. Leonetti had been, the next morning brought with it something even worse. I received another call from the school. I had become used to them now; Will's counselor and I were becoming friends.

"Hello, Mrs. Perry," I began.

"This is not Mrs. Perry," said a stern voice. "My name is Margaret Kruger. I run the counseling staff here at Pine Crest."

"Oh, I'm sorry. How are you, Ms. Kruger?"

"Not good. It has come to my attention that your son, William, has been coming to our offices on a regular basis."

"Oh, yes. As Mrs. Perry knows, our family is going through a difficult period, and he's having a hard time."

"Mr. Dylan, a hard time is an understatement. It appears to me that your child cannot function properly."

"Wait a second," I said, offended, "he's doing his best. The situation at home is very difficult. His mother has been sick for several weeks now." Once again, I was avoiding the truth, concerned that the stigma surrounding mental illness would invite more scrutiny.

"Sir, in cases like these we call DCF, the Department of Children and Families," she snapped. I didn't know much about the organization, but I did know that she had just threatened to get the government involved. "When we hear that a child is scared of his home, unable to deal with his parents, then we have to take action."

"My son is not scared of his home. Unable to deal with his parents? Are you kidding me? When he comes to your office, it's because he wants to call me for support."

"Sir, your son is missing class on a regular basis. He is clearly crying for help."

"Yes—he's crying *to me* for help! How would DCF help? Would they take him away from me? That would be the worst thing in the world they could do!" I was becoming scared and angry.

"We'll let DCF make that decision."

"No, we won't. You are not going to call the government!"

"Mr. Dylan, you need to listen to me—"

"No, you need to listen to me, Ms. Kruger!" I caught myself and took a deep breath. Fighting this woman was not a winning strategy. I started again more calmly.

"Ms. Kruger, with all due respect to you and the responsibilities of your job, we have a loving home. My son is a good kid, and he's always been a great student. We are dealing with a major health crisis, and he is scared. But I have worked with Mrs. Perry to find a counselor to help him with his anxiety."

I paused; she seemed to be listening, so I continued. "On Monday, he's seeing Matthew Brown, someone that Mrs. Perry recommended. Please give him some time with my son. If, after a couple of weeks, things don't improve, then you can call DCF."

Silence. I could tell that she was considering it.

"Ms. Kruger, please. My wife's sickness has been difficult for everyone. But my kids and I, we need to stay together. It's crucial that we stay together." I was almost breaking into sobs.

"Okay, Mr. Dylan," she replied, a gentler tone to her voice. "I'll speak with Mrs. Perry. We'll give it another week, but we need to see improvement, okay?"

"Yes, thank you," I gushed. "Thank you for your under-standing."

As we moved into the weekend, I realized that Saturday and Sunday had lost their magic. Our house was no longer a place to relax. Mia was always upset, and the kids and I remained tense. Mia left dinners early, which at least gave the kids a chance to play their favorite game with their uncle. One of those nights, Will asked, "Uncle Luke, what's the most dangerous job you've ever had?"

"I know that one!" I chimed in. "You've seen that pic-ture where Uncle Luke is luring the crocodile out of the water?"

"Ah, yeah!" crowed Luke. "I almost forgot about that one." He looked wistful, like he was back standing by that muddy lagoon. Then his expression changed abruptly. "But nah, Patricio, that's not it."

He had our attention; what could be worse than danc-ing up close with gigantic, man-eating crocodiles?

"Mira," he began, "there was this one time I was in Costa Rica. Pretty country, Costa Rica. They got all kinds of terrain, yeah? They got these beaches on the coasts and these huge rain forests in the middle.

"So, I know this dude, and he knows I can dive, sí?" he continued. "And he knows this other guy and . . . *pa pa pa, pe pe pe* . . . I wind up on this crew. Actually, I was leading the crew. And there was this forest within the rain forest, you know? Mira, these trees were called *cocobolo*, and they were old and fully mature." Luke made a motion with his hand, like he was pointing out something tall.

"And cocobolo, it's like rosewood, yeah? And I tell you, that shit's hella expensive," he said. Again, I flashed him the *no swearing* look. He nodded apologetically.

"So, they hired us to harvest these trees, this forest of cocobolo trees. The only thing is, in that particular area, the forest had been flooded. All the trees were underwater!"

The kids were wearing the same puzzled expression that I was. "Luke, how do you harvest trees that are underwater?" I asked.

"Ahh, that's what made it so dangerous, Patricio!" he cried, pointing at me. "They gave us these chain saws, see? But they were underwater chain saws. The water was already cloudy, but when you took those chain saws and started cutting into the trees—yo, you couldn't see a damn thing!"

I had never heard of underwater chain saws, but Luke wasn't the type to make up stories; he didn't need to.

"And I had these guys on my crew. I was the *jefe*, but these guys were out of control, man. *Loco.* You never knew where they were. I'd be down there in my dive suit all day—hours, bro—just sawing these trees, without being able to see shit, and knowing these guys were all around me, cutting away. And when you finally cut through a tree, it would float to the surface. You had to watch it because if that tree knocked out your regulator and you got spun around, you wouldn't know which way was up." He paused, shuddering. "That was some scary shit."

I threw him another accusatory look, but he wasn't paying attention. He was back under the water with his team of wild lumberjacks.

"Yo, it paid well, though," he smirked, his eyes refocusing on us. "It paid *really* well."

And that was the way we spent our weekend. Luke, the kids, and I enjoyed our time together, and Mia maintained her distance.

On Monday, I picked up Will from school and took him to his first appointment with Matthew Brown. It was immediately apparent that Matthew specialized in working with kids. He quickly introduced us to his sidekick, a lovable golden retriever named Tanner. Matthew's office was inviting, with Florida State paraphernalia everywhere. Will was a college-football fan, and the two immediately bonded over talk of upcoming games.

After the session, they both thought that establishing a regular schedule of appointments would be helpful, and I jumped at their suggestion. The drive home didn't reveal much, however. Will was reluctant to disclose what they had discussed and stared pensively out the window at the palm trees passing by. But the next morning, Matthew called as I was driving into work.

"Hi, Pat," he started. "My approach is to treat conversations confidentially. However, you should know that I will always alert a parent if I am seriously concerned about their child."

"Okay . . . ," I replied uncertainly.

"Will is a delightful kid. I'm not worried about him, but I wanted to give you some thoughts on the situation. Obviously, what's going on with your wife has triggered his anxiety."

"I know. We're all worried about her."

"Right, but Will is actually okay with his mother's sickness. That's not what has him skipping school."

"What? I don't understand."

"Here's the thing," said Matthew, "and don't take this the wrong way. Will has already given up on his mom. It's not that he doesn't want her to get better, or that he doesn't think that she will, but he doesn't understand it."

I waited, still not following.

"As far as he's concerned, he has already lost one parent. That's why he's always calling and texting you. He wants to be sure that he doesn't lose you, too."

Sudden clarity flooded my thinking. It was so obvious once Matthew explained it.

"He told you that?"

"Well, not in so many words, but yeah, that's what's going on here."

"Can you help him, give him ways to deal with it?"

"Yes, of course. His anxiety is normal for this kind of situation. We have a lot of tools that he can use. We already started using some of them yesterday."

Hanging up, I exhaled slowly and thought about Will. Separation anxiety made perfect sense. I smiled, grateful that we had identified the right person for him. My mind turned immediately to Jamie, reaffirming the need to find someone for her, too. But my first priority was securing Mia's new psychiatrist.

Later that day, Mia and I went to our first meeting with Dr. Rojas. The waiting room had all the familiar trappings: the friendly receptionist, the leather sofa, the soothing white noise.

We sat in silent anticipation for several minutes, and then Dr. Rojas emerged from the hallway. He greeted us warmly, shaking Mia's hand first. He was short in stature, with kind eyes and a gentle disposition. He moved confidently, and I later learned that he had served in the army. More than anything, he radiated serenity.

Mia and I settled into a couch against one wall of his large, well-appointed office. Rather than sit behind his desk,

Dr. Rojas took a chair next us. "So, how is *Mia* today?" he asked, smiling broadly as he emphasized her name.

Mia summarized the stages of her illness. Dr. Rojas asked clarifying questions periodically, but he mostly listened. He did pose the standard queries about hearing voices and having delusions. To my relief, Mia answered them honestly, acknowledging that she still had paranoid thoughts. I spoke only when he asked about current medications. Mia couldn't seem to name them on her own.

"Seroquel wouldn't be my drug of choice," he stated, "but I'm hesitant to switch now, given that things are finally under control. So, let's stay on the current protocol. But let's also add one baby aspirin per day."

I must have given him a strange look, because Dr. Rojas added, "Pat, your wife has had what amounts to a heart attack, but the organ that was affected was not her heart. It was her brain. Unfortunately, we don't know nearly as much about the brain, but I guarantee you that she has swelling. Taking baby aspirin won't hurt, and it might just help."

I thought about his analogy. "So, Dr. Rojas, do you think this could be a onetime thing? Like maybe we can prevent another heart attack from happening?"

"I do think that. I agree with your first diagnosis, that this was brief reactive psychosis. The stress from Mia's job, and the disrupted sleep that followed, was too much for her brain to handle. It has suffered greatly, and it will take time to heal. But once it does, she'll be fine."

He turned to Mia. "You'll have to find ways to cope with your anxiety," he instructed, "but I don't think you have a chronic condition. It doesn't align with the rest of your history."

We spent over an hour with Dr. Rojas. He was thorough and patient, and I hoped that Mia liked him as much as I did. It was a good sign when she took the lead in arranging the next appointment.

Normally, after a meeting of that gravity, Mia and I would have spent more time talking about it, but now a silent car ride was all that followed. By this point, Mia had been out of the crisis center for a week. Each day, I kept hoping that she would start acting more like herself; and each day, I remained disappointed.

One challenge when interacting with Mia was that she had become hyperfocused on the exact words being used in an exchange. And if you weren't precise, it would infuriate her. We might be out walking the dog, and she would ask, "Do you know if the front door is unlocked?"

I would respond, without much thought, "Yeah, I think it's open."

"The front door is not open, Pat," she would retort, giving me a nasty look. "I can see it from here." And then she would be mad at me for hours. The correct answer would have been, "Yes, the front door is unlocked."

She was vigilant in listening to each word to be sure she was processing everything correctly; she didn't know if she could trust her own thoughts. But trying to speak so accurately for even a half hour was exhausting. It was impossible not to resort to common idioms, no matter how hard we tried.

In addition, we started to notice how many everyday expressions referred to mental illness. I would be talking to Mia and say something like, "Sorry I'm late, the traffic was insane." And then I'd feel terrible about it. Or I would quip: "I wish the weather would cool down; it's driving me crazy." I hesitated to even open my mouth.

Another challenge was that her short-term memory was suffering badly. All of her medications compromised retention, especially the Ativan and Restoril. She couldn't remember things that had happened literally ten minutes prior. Coupled with her paranoia, this meant that she continually thought we were playing tricks on her.

Mia was like Dory from *Finding Nemo*. Given how quickly she forgot things, her phone became an essential part of her existence. She was constantly entering reminders and adding to her to-do lists. One day, she arranged to call our sister-in-law Jen at 6:15 p.m. But instead of entering it as a onetime event, she must have accidentally hit the "every day" button. So, Mia would see an alarm pop up at 6:15 p.m. every night and call Jen, not remembering that she had already spoken with her the prior day. This went on for weeks.

The paranoia was another issue. As I've said, Mia saved that for me. It wasn't as bad as when she was psychotic, but anything out of the ordinary would throw her off. A stranger walking her dog down the street? She was plotting against us. Someone checking the sprinkler system for the house next door? He was a potential thief casing the place for a robbery.

Driving was yet another problem. Because Mia was on so much medication, Dr. Martinez had instructed us not to let her use the car. Luke or I had to chaperone her everywhere, and she hated it. She resented being continuously under our watch and wanted her freedom back.

Things were hardest at the end of the day, when we were alone in our room. Before she became sick, nighttime was when we connected as a couple. But now, we were two strangers, ignoring each other while brushing our teeth. I was afraid to ask what she was thinking, fearful that any prodding might upset her more.

Before her illness, Mia and I had never fought, but now we regularly turned out the lights with a cloud of unresolved conflict hanging heavily over us. I became accustomed to lying in the dark, wondering if my partner would ever recover. I felt an overwhelming sense of loneliness, like a single parent whose spouse had left or died.

At last, the day came for our dreaded appointment with the treatment center to discuss Mia's rape allegations. We didn't meet at the crisis center. Instead, they sent us to a conference room in one of the adjacent buildings. It was a typical industrial meeting space with plastic chairs collected around a cheap table. Fluorescent lights buzzed overhead.

Three women were waiting for us when we arrived. I recognized two of them from my visits, but the third was new. She seemed to be in charge, calling the meeting to order and reviewing the reasons for it. She then asked Mia to provide the details of her complaint.

Mia talked about being treated badly, pushed around and held down on various occasions. This wasn't surprising; I had witnessed a couple of these instances myself. Mia kept looking my way, expecting me to jump in and start attacking the staff, but I couldn't do it. From what I had seen, the folks in the crisis center did what was necessary. I was thankful for their help.

In the end, the meeting didn't amount to much. Mia never accused anyone of rape, and I remained silent. When she realized that I wasn't going to participate, she ran out of steam. The woman in charge asked Mia to sign a few forms, essentially testifying that the meeting had taken place. The whole thing lasted less than thirty minutes.

Back in the car, Mia was furious. "I can't believe you took their side!" she hissed. "You're supposed to be supporting me!"

"What are you talking about? Of course I support you."

"It didn't look like it in there, Pat! You didn't say a word."

"I only know what I saw when I visited you, and I didn't see any crimes committed. I would certainly have spoken up if I had."

Mia seethed quietly in resentment. When we arrived home, she went straight to our room and shut the door. I felt bad knowing that she was so upset, but it would have been wrong to accuse the GTC of malfeasance. Besides, I was becoming acclimated to Mia's bitterness.

That weekend passed in much the same way as the previous one. Luke, the kids, and I lived as normally as possible, and Mia locked herself away. On a positive note, Will hadn't texted or called from school on Friday. He had seen Matthew only twice, but already things were improving.

"Hey," I said, stopping by his room and trying to sound as casual as possible, "seems like things are going better for you?"

"Yeah, thanks. They are."

"So, Matthew is helping?"

"He is. He gave me several things to try. One was to write down all the stuff that was worrying me."

"Really?"

"Yeah, he said just write it all down whenever I started to worry. And once it's written down, I don't have to keep running it over and over in my head."

"Wow, does that work? I never would have thought of that."

"Me neither, but the more I do it, the better I feel," he said. "So, I'm going to keep doing it."

On Sunday morning, I was surprised when Mia approached me. We hadn't spoken more than two words since the GTC visit. She told me that she felt one of her migraines starting and wanted to know if she could take her prescription for it, a drug called Relpax. I had no idea, so I called Dr. Rojas. He advised me that it shouldn't be a problem.

It made me nervous, but Mia's migraines were debilitating. It was almost impossible not to use the medication.

On Monday at work, I began to feel optimistic. Mia was constantly mad at me, but at least she was stabilized. And we continued to find great therapists, having met both Dr. Rojas and Matthew Brown recently. I missed the healthy Mia terribly, but I firmly believed that time would bring her back to us.

Therefore, it was deeply unsettling when she shut the door to our bedroom as soon as I arrived home from work that night.

"Pat, I need to tell you something," she whispered. "There are people listening outside the windows."

"What are you talking about, babe?"

She gave me the sign to be quiet, putting a finger to her mouth and then pointing at the nearest window. "They've got hidden listening devices," she murmured. "They don't want us to know."

I was used to her paranoia, but this was different. When Mia had paranoid thoughts, she divulged her suspicions to me. She solicited my feedback, and she would listen intently to my answers. But at the moment, she was fully vested in her belief that we were being stalked.

A month earlier, her bizarre warning would have scared me, but I found myself more puzzled than anything. She remained on huge amounts of Seroquel; by all accounts, she should be gradually improving. My thoughts immediately went to the migraine medication. Could it have interfered with her recovery?

Within ten minutes, I had comforted Mia to the best of my ability, escaped to the driveway, and called Dr. Rojas. He thought it possible that Mia was suffering a short setback, and that it would improve with sleep. He instructed me to give her an extra dose of Ativan right away and keep her under surveillance, assuring me that the Relpax shouldn't have caused any problems. Fortunately, we had a meeting scheduled with him the following afternoon, where he could conduct a full assessment.

We stayed in our bedroom. I gave her the Ativan first and then, about ninety minutes later, the rest of her medication. She fell asleep easily. When she did, I pulled Luke aside to update him on the situation.

I left for work before Mia woke up the next morning, hoping that her sleeping in was a positive sign. However, I soon received a call from Luke. I was in a meeting at the time and excused myself to answer.

"Dude, Mia is on another *planet*," he said, emphasizing the last word.

"What do you mean? How is she behaving?"

"She's trippin', bro. What she's saying doesn't make any sense, all paranoid and crazy and shit. It's like you described it, man. She's gone."

My heart sank. "Okay, just keep her in the house and keep her safe. I'll be home soon."

Hanging up, I reached out to the wall for support. I felt like someone running an endless race whose legs have finally given out. All the surreal moments over the past three weeks began racing through my mind.

How can this be happening to us? I thought, fighting back tears. *What the hell is going on?*

Rather than a short setback, this seemed like a major relapse. The tears were for Mia. I was doing everything possible but still failing her. The medication wasn't working; the expert advice was leading us nowhere.

Arriving home, my worst fears were realized. Mia's psychosis had progressed from paranoid delusions to the other symptoms I knew all too well. "Concrete thinking" was back, where she misinterpreted things that were said by taking them literally. "Centers of reference" had also returned, where she believed that songs on the radio were written specifically for her.

And, once again, she was seeing clues to mysterious puzzles everywhere.

12.

THE RESURGENCE

The Cure
"Pictures of You"
4:07–4:38

My brother, Brad, was the best man at our wedding, and he gave a thoughtful toast, essentially marveling at Mia's kindness and wondering how I ever persuaded her to marry me. It was funny and moving, and he delivered it perfectly. He was a tough act to follow.

Fortunately, I had been preparing for months. Unbeknownst to Mia, I had secretly written a toast in Spanish. A native speaker helped me practice it. By our reception, I could recite it word for word fluently. I followed my brother to the stage when he finished; everyone expected English to come next.

"Antes de empezar, quiero decir unas palabras en el primer idioma de Mia." Translated, this meant: "Before I start, I want to say a few words in Mia's first language." The speech included lots of references to Miami and fishing, too. The audience, half of whom were Cuban, roared with approval. They were impressed, I think, because it lasted over five minutes. They all loved it, especially Mark and Luke. I could hear them hollering from the tables below.

After the Spanish toast, I gave one in English. It talked about how I used to dream about the right girl for me. I made reference to one of my favorite movies, *Butch Cassidy and the Sundance Kid*. There's a scene where Robert Redford describes what he is looking for in a partner: "I'm not picky. As long as she's smart, pretty, and sweet, and gentle, and tender, and refined, and lovely, and carefree . . ." He walks away, his voice trailing off as he keeps listing adjectives.

That was how it felt when I was younger, like I was searching for someone too perfect to be real. But then I met Mia, and she was everything that I had dreamed about. Some people might have felt embarrassed or uncomfortable, standing on a stage and admitting these things. I felt invincible, proudly facing the crowd of people that meant so much to us.

But there was another memory that meant more to me. It came after the seriousness of the ceremony and the clamor of the reception.

We left early on Monday morning for our honeymoon. We were looking forward to a week in the Caribbean together. But as I sat on the plane, I realized that it was way more than that: we were looking forward to a lifetime together.

And it hit me—I would never be alone again. Sure, we might be separated for a few days here and there, but Mia was my eternal companion. This beautiful, talented, and kindhearted person would always be there for me. Of course, we would go through difficult times, but we'd go through them together. We would always have each other to lean on.

I thought that at the time, anyway.

***

Mia was fully psychotic again. Before too long, we were sitting in Dr. Rojas's waiting room. The white noise was helpful, as it captured and held her attention. As we waited, I kept thinking about our first visit. It had only been a week, but the situation had deteriorated dramatically.

"So, how is *Mia* today?" asked Dr. Rojas after we had settled into his office.

Mia didn't answer his question and focused instead on counting the ceiling tiles in his office. She kept repeating that the number eight must have something to do with it.

Dr. Rojas tried a couple of times to get her on track, but it was no use. "Okay, Mia," said Dr. Rojas, interrupting her, "could you please wait here in my office? I have some samples of a new medication we might like to try." Turning to me, he said, "Pat, could you come with me? I'll need some help."

"Um, sure," I said. Dr. Rojas held the door, closing it as he followed me through.

"Pat, my God!" he exclaimed. "What happened? She's so much worse than last week!"

"I don't know. Things changed so quickly, that's why I thought it might have something to do with the Relpax."

"No, no, the Relpax couldn't have caused this reaction."

We were right outside his office. I wondered if Mia might be able to hear us.

"Are you sure she has been taking the Seroquel?" he asked.

"I don't have any reason to believe that she hasn't. I'm usually there when she takes it." This was true, although I hadn't made a point of studying her closely while she did.

"I've never seen anything like this," admitted Dr. Rojas after a pause, "such a dramatic change when on such high doses of Seroquel for so long. It shouldn't be happening." He paused again, his mouth folding down into a slight frown. "Pat, if I were treating this from the beginning, I would have put Mia on Zyprexa."

"Zyprexa?"

"It's a much older drug than Seroquel, used to treat bipolar and schizophrenia. We have much more data on its effectiveness. I've had very good success with it when dealing with psychosis."

"Will it be a problem if she takes it with the Seroquel?"

"It shouldn't cause an adverse reaction, but she will be heavily medicated." I could tell he was thinking it through as we talked.

"She's already heavily medicated," I sighed.

"I can't bring down the Seroquel too quickly, that could cause problems, but it doesn't seem to be the right drug for her. People respond to these medications in all different ways."

"You have way more experience with this stuff than I do," I said. "But I would agree with you, the Seroquel doesn't seem to be working. I'm okay with making a change if you think we should."

Dr. Rojas looked at me. "Thank you for your trust, Pat," he said evenly. "We are going to wean Mia off Seroquel and start her on Zyprexa. Come with me."

I followed him down the hallway. He opened a closet, and I saw boxes of medications piled high. "These are Zyprexa samples." He opened a plastic bag and threw little purple packets inside. "They won't approve the Zyprexa prescription until the Seroquel runs out. These samples will allow us to start on it immediately."

He handed me the bag. "I'll write down specific instructions on how to administer the medications. It's going to be very important that you follow my directions exactly."

"Okay," I said nervously. We were mixing strong, brain-altering pharmaceuticals. What kind of effect would that have on Mia?

"Good," said Dr. Rojas, his eyes steady. "And Pat, you have to make sure that Mia takes the medication. Watch her take it, every single time."

When we arrived home, I had carefully detailed instructions on how to manage Mia's medications. Dr. Rojas wanted to precisely titrate the Zyprexa and Seroquel, increasing the first while slowly decreasing the second. With pills everywhere, the counter of my dresser looked like a pharmacy.

Mia took her first dose of Zyprexa immediately. I gave it to her reluctantly, apprehensive about loading up on so many psychotropic drugs. But I trusted Dr. Rojas, and the Seroquel was clearly failing.

Luke and I took turns watching Mia the rest of the day. I stayed with her initially, making sure that she didn't become worse with the new medication. Then he took a shift so I could make dinner and help the kids with homework. When I checked back in with Luke, he and Mia were secluded in our bedroom.

She was in the bathroom, but he looked up from the bed. He was lying down and fiddling with his phone. Although he wouldn't sleep on a mattress, he didn't mind relaxing on one.

"Yo, Patricio," he said, "she's been good for the past ten minutes or so."

"Really?"

"Yeah, bro. Before that, nah, she was all confused . . . *pa pa pa, pe pe pe* . . . rambling here and there. But then she became more coherent."

"Thanks, Cubano. I'll manage things from here."

I took his spot on the bed. Closing my eyes, I tried to enjoy the brief silence, but it wasn't possible. My body was taut, prepared for battle. After a couple of minutes, Mia came out of the bathroom.

"Hi, Pat," she said. I opened my eyes; she sounded normal.

"Hi," I replied. "How are you doing?"

She let out a big sigh, then sat on the bed next to me. "What is going on?" she asked wearily. "None of this feels right."

"No, it doesn't," I admitted.

"Why have I been treating you so badly? I've been so mean to you."

I didn't answer.

"I'm so sorry, babe." She put her hand on my leg. "This must be horrible for you."

I couldn't believe it—Mia seemed suddenly cured! I sat up quickly.

"Um, yeah, it hasn't been great," I replied, "but it's okay."

With sincere tenderness in her voice, she said, "I'm so sorry."

We sat looking at each other for a moment. "Mia, is that . . . is that really you?" I asked, staring into her eyes. And I saw it; I saw that connection I had been craving for so long.

"Yeah, Pat, it's me."

I kissed her and wrapped her in an eager hug. She reciprocated the embrace. I tried desperately to enjoy the moment, but my mind was racing. Could the Zyprexa have worked so quickly? It didn't seem possible.

"What are we going to do?" she asked, trying to pull away.

"I don't know, whatever we have to do," I responded, unwilling to let her go. Could she be better? Was the nightmare over?

"What about the kids? Are they okay?"

"They're okay," I promised, finally releasing her.

She sat back, smiling weakly. I still had her hands in mine, holding them in my lap. I didn't want her to move, didn't want the moment to end. But less than a minute later, she stood up and walked across the room.

"There's got to be some reason for it," she said.

No, no, don't go looking for reasons, I begged silently.

"If we can figure out the reason, we can find a solution."

No, don't worry about that now. Stay with me!

"Maybe if we just go backward . . ." And then it was over, as quickly as it had started. She was trapped again in psychosis, swirling through disjointed ideas.

At the time, it was absolute torture. But in days to come, that exchange became a source of inspiration. I knew that my Mia was somewhere in there, ensnared inside a spiraling brain.

After she fell sleep, I received a text from her cousin Alex. I hadn't spoken to him in over a week, but I knew that Mark was keeping him updated. Rather than text back, I called.

"It's been tough, Alex," I said after he answered. "She did have a brief moment of clarity tonight, but it didn't last long."

"Dude, I guarantee you she stopped taking the Seroquel," he blurted out. "There's no other way she could be psychotic again."

"That's what her psychiatrist thought, too," I said, "but I don't see how that could be possible. Either I've been there or Luke has been there every time we've given it to her."

"You don't see it because you haven't dealt with mentally ill patients before. They hate the way the medication makes them feel. They get really good at faking it."

"Faking it?"

"They put the pills in their mouth and pretend to swallow them, but then, when you aren't looking, they spit them out."

"I don't know about that," I replied. "She took Relpax for her migraine on Sunday. Isn't it possible that it triggered some kind of relapse?"

I could hear him looking up the details in his reference guide.

"No, that shouldn't have caused it," he said. "Pat, trust me on this. You need to go buy a safe. You need to do it tonight."

"A safe? What are you talking about?"

"Here's the next phase of this; I've seen it a million times. If you leave the medication on the counter, you'll go to give her a dose and she'll say, 'It's okay, I've already taken it.' And you won't know if she has or not. You'll be scared to give her too much, so you'll let it go."

"You mean, I should lock up the medication so I know exactly when it has been accessed?"

"Exactly," he agreed. "Even small changes to the dose can set things off. You can't let that happen. You have to know for sure that she has taken it. And you have to know exactly how much she has taken and when. Another thing, when you give her the medication, watch her take it. Make her open her mouth afterward and show you that the pills are gone."

"Jesus, man, that will really make her mad."

"Who cares if she's mad? The only thing that matters is that she takes the medication. Takes it at the right dose."

"Yeah, I guess so. You're right."

"I'm definitely right," he said. "There's no way that little Mia could be psychotic again on that much Seroquel. No way."

A half hour later, I was standing in a brightly lit aisle of Walmart, evaluating the various options for safes. I chose a medium-size one, big enough to hold the plastic bottles but small enough to fit next to my dresser. Back home, I programmed the lock and arranged the medicine inside. I showed it to Luke, too, bringing him up to speed on Alex's advice.

I stayed home from work the next day. After she woke, I gave Mia the day's first round of medication. She didn't notice the safe, but she was not pleased when I asked to see that she had swallowed the pills. She finally complied when I said it was her cousin Alex's idea: opening her mouth, sticking out her tongue, and casting a withering stare afterward.

Her psychosis continued all day, but the pattern was different. She had dramatic swings in behavior. She would be fairly reserved for a while, never quite approaching the clarity of the previous night but acting almost normal. This might last twenty minutes or so. And then abruptly she'd be raving again.

Luke and I continued swapping out responsibility. Keeping her contained to the bedroom became impossible. She refused to stay in one spot and wasn't easily distracted. But she didn't try to run away, and she didn't feel threatened, either.

I left in the afternoon to take Will to another session with his counselor. I picked Jamie up at the bus stop along the way, wanting to keep her out of the house. Neither of the kids knew that Mia had relapsed, and I wasn't sure how to break the news.

Will met with Matthew while Jamie and I read together in the waiting room. Once we were all in the car, I decided it couldn't wait any longer.

"Guys," I said, turning down the radio, "I wanted to talk to you about Mom again."

They didn't reply, so I continued. "I know her illness has been really hard on everyone."

I waited a second; they were listening.

"And, as we have learned, her illness comes and goes. Sometimes she acts really weird, and that's when the sickness is messing with her thoughts. She can't think straight. And other times she acts mean, not like her usual self. And that's because of her medication. Remember when we talked about that?"

"Yes," said Will in a low voice.

"Yes," echoed Jamie.

"Okay, well, I wanted to let you know that Mom is acting really weird again," I said. "It started yesterday. But even though she might be acting funny, she's still the same Mom inside. It's her sickness that we're seeing, not Mom. We just need to remember that and try to be as patient as we can. Think you can do that?"

"Yes," whispered Will again.

"Yes," repeated Jamie, just as quietly.

"Thanks," I said, "and if things get too uncomfortable, you can always excuse yourself and go to your room. Or you can come to me or Uncle Luke if you want to talk."

"Okay," they both said, barely audible.

"Hey, you two!" I said with false cheer. "Mom isn't dying! She's going to get better. I know it is taking longer than any of us thought, but she's going to get better."

They both kind of nodded their heads like they agreed, and I decided to stop there. I turned the radio back up, but a sense of anticipation filled the air. None of us knew what to expect when we arrived home.

Mia was out by the pool with Luke when we walked in, so Will and Jamie retreated to their rooms. When dinner was ready, everyone came into the kitchen to get their food, and it looked like we might have a normal meal—until Mia appeared.

She was clearly agitated and in her own world. Mumbling under her breath, she made her way to the table and then started walking around it, studying the plates and silverware.

"No, this isn't right," she said, grabbing Luke's plate. He sat looking at Mia while she continued circling the table, holding his food. The rest of us had paused and were watching her now, too.

Mia put Luke's dish down at a different spot and stood looking at it. "No, no," she muttered, picking it up again. Then she looked over at Will. "You sit here," she ordered, pointing down at a chair. "Right here."

Will glanced over at me; I shrugged.

"Come on," Mia said. "Don't be afraid. This is your place."

Will sat. Mia continued to circle, finally putting Luke's plate down and instructing him to switch chairs. This went on for five minutes, with Mia concentrating hard to unravel the correct arrangement of seats.

Then she began to rearrange the silverware. She was picking up people's forks, believing they had to be paired with certain plates. I finally stepped in.

"Okay, that's all, babe," I said, taking the silverware out of her hands. "You don't need to worry about any of this right now." The kids had seen their mom acting bizarrely enough.

Mia stared at me, a nervous glaze to her eyes. I was keenly aware of my actions and my tone; I knew the kids were watching.

"C'mon," I said tenderly, "let's get you some food." I put my arms around her shoulders and led her over to the kitchen, hoping that she wouldn't react negatively.

Once she had her food to focus on, Mia was better. She sat silently for a while, but I could tell that she was frustrated. The kids were talking about school, but she wasn't able to follow the conversation. I suggested that she and I return to the bedroom.

For the rest of the night, the illness displayed a pattern similar to the one we had seen during the day. At times, she was calm and almost coherent, but then she would become extremely confused and paranoid. One common thread ran through it all: she became upset every time we forced her to show us that she had swallowed the medication.

On Thursday morning, Luke offered to watch Mia for the day and update me as needed, but I decided to stay home again from work. I wanted a firsthand view of her condition.

As the day progressed, her psychosis became more belligerent; she was especially quick-tempered with me. At this point, she was losing her phone every twenty minutes. Mia asked us to help her look for it at least fifteen times that day. After we found it, she would usually accuse us of stealing it. "If we had stolen it, why would we help you find it?" I asked the first time it happened, hoping to defuse the situation. Unfortunately, she thought I was teasing her. All it did was widen the divide between us.

And even though the devil hadn't shown up again, Mia was exhibiting signs of intense religiousness. This was not like her; she had never been preachy. Now, she was listening nonstop to Christian radio at high volumes, usually turning it up even louder when I walked into the room.

In the afternoon, Mia continued cycling through degrees of psychosis, becoming more hostile during the worst phases. I was worried about the crescendo; my gut told me that we were headed toward an untenable situation. Alarmed, I texted Dr. Rojas. He instructed me to slow the rate of increase of Zyprexa.

Luke and I kept Mia away from the kids that night; she was too unpredictable and antagonistic. Finally, I was on the last shift of the night with her. She was talking with her mom on the phone, in our bedroom. It was during one of her lucid phases, and their conversation sounded quasi-normal. Not realizing that Mia was watching, I went over to the safe to assemble her last dose of medication for the day.

"Wow, look at this!" I heard Mia say to Lucia. "Pat has a safe here, Mom. A safe!"

I glanced back at Mia.

"What's the safe for, Pat?"

"It's just so I can keep track of the medication," I answered, trying to remain calm.

"Keep track of the medication? What are you going to do, lose it?" she sneered.

I was kneeling on the floor by the safe, not sure how to respond.

"I think he's taking the medication now, too," she said to Lucia. "He's guarding it for himself. That's smart, Pat. It's about time you started taking the medication. You need it!"

"It's another one of Alex's suggestions," I explained, ignoring her accusation.

"Oh, Alex has a lot of great suggestions!" thundered Mia. "He's the reason you and Luke don't trust me to take the pills by myself."

"He said it was important that you take them as instructed." My heart was beating faster.

"Haven't I been doing that, Pat?" she screamed, pulling the phone away from her cheek. "Haven't I been taking the medication for weeks now?"

"Yes."

"For weeks! And now you have a safe? Where'd the safe come from, Pat? Tell me the truth!"

I wanted to scream, too. How many times would she ask me about the truth?

"Mom, listen to this!" she howled, putting the phone back to her ear. "Pat doesn't trust me to take the pills. He makes me open my mouth and show that I swallowed them, like a little kid!"

I couldn't hear what Lucia was saying, but it made Mia snarl. "Have you been talking to Alex, too? Or did Pat tell you to say that?"

She paused to listen, a disgusted look on her face.

"Fine!" she snapped. "I've got to go. Here, you can talk to Pat."

Mia threw her phone at me. Catching it, I kept an eye on Mia as I spoke, "Hi, Lucia."

"Oh, Pat, we are very sorry that you have to go through this," she said. I could hear the distress in her voice.

Mia walked into the bathroom.

"It's okay," I said. "Um, I really hate to do this, but I have to let you go."

Hanging up, I stood listening for a second. I couldn't tell what Mia was doing, but at least I knew where she was. When she came back out, I had the medication ready, along with a glass of water. To my surprise, she stomped over to me in a huff and, glaring at me, grabbed the pills.

It always took her a while to swallow the medications; she had to go one pill at a time. And with the addition of Zyprexa, she was now taking eight pills three times a day. But she started swigging them down, without saying a word. When she finished, she turned to me, opened her mouth, and stuck out her tongue. "Happy now?"

She ignored me the rest of the night. After she fell asleep, I snuck out to review the day with Luke. He agreed that Mia's condition was becoming explosive.

"I'm afraid we're getting to the point where she'll have to go back to the crisis center," I confessed, "and I hate it. I mean, they're good people, but if she goes back there, we lose all control over the situation."

"Fuck it, then," said Luke. "Don't send her back."

"They keep her safe in there, though."

"We can keep her safe here. You and me, bro. We'll make sure she can't get out . . . Lockdown."

I considered his idea. I could keep Dr. Rojas fully informed of her condition. He could act as our in-house psychiatrist. I would have to do something with the kids, though; no way could they be part of it.

"I don't know," I said, still undecided. "Last time she was in there it took a week to get out. We can't keep her locked down in the house for a week. We've got the kids."

"Then let's take her over to my parents' house," suggested Luke. "They come here and watch the kids; we take her over there. Whatever shit happens, we handle it. Mark would be down."

The idea was tempting. Luke and Mark were the ideal partners for a scheme like that. But two things made it unrealistic. First, I didn't want to be away from the kids for even a few days. Will clearly needed me around, and I guessed that Jamie did, too. Second, the ordeal would be difficult for Mia. Even the three-hour trip to her parents' house would be traumatic.

"It's a good thought, and maybe it comes to that," I said, "but for now, let's brace ourselves for the weekend. I'll get the kids out of the house after school tomorrow, and hopefully things will improve by Sunday."

"You got it, Patricio." He nodded his head in support. I felt more confident knowing that Luke had my back.

The illness was gaining in strength; I didn't want to face it alone.

13.

THE WORST NIGHT EVER

Broken Bells
"The High Road"
1:37–1:48

Mia landed her first job the month after she graduated from the PA program. I was stunned how quickly she had offers. She accepted a position with a sole practitioner. Dr. Ted Bailey ran a popular pediatrics office about five minutes from our Houston apartment. He was a family man, with three daughters and a supportive wife, and he spent too much time at the office. Hiring Mia would allow him to take a day off every now and then.

Both Mia and I really liked Dr. Bailey. He was an experienced and caring physician who invested a lot of time in his patients. He also had a dry, self-deprecating sense of humor that made him immediately likable. He made the ideal mentor.

Within a few weeks, Mia was seeing patients on her own. It had only been three years, but she had already accomplished the goal she had set for herself after college.

She was helping people and doing everything a doctor could do.

I hadn't set any real goals for myself at graduation, other than to pay off student loans. I hadn't enjoyed working at the investment bank, and my finance job in Houston was interesting but not in pursuit of any long-term objective. When it came to my career, I was floundering.

Mia encouraged me to consider graduate school. It would allow me to think carefully about what I wanted to do with my life. Professionally, I had no sense of purpose, which was especially clear when juxtaposed with the fulfillment Mia received from her work. I began applying to business programs.

Meanwhile, as they worked together, it became apparent that Dr. Bailey prized his relationship with Mia. She was diligent and thorough with his patients, and he trusted her.

However, Mia and I faced a difficult decision nine months into her dream job. I had been accepted to a few business schools, including Harvard, but my attendance would require a move. That meant saying goodbye to Dr. Bailey.

"Of course, I'd hate to leave," Mia said, "but we need to consider our long-term goals. We don't have any relatives here, and we've always said that being close to family is important. And if we go back to Harvard, odds are that you'll have the flexibility to get a job somewhere near family, whether that be in Florida or back in Chicago." She included the Midwest for my sake; Mia's dream was to ultimately settle within driving distance of Miami.

"Yes, that's true," I replied.

"Then, Pat, it seems pretty clear: we have to go." After finding her perfect position, she was willing to give it up for me and our future together.

We shared dinner with the Baileys a few times that year. Mia and I enjoyed spending time with their family. The Bailey girls were middle and elementary school kids, with little frames and big personalities. I enjoyed watching Mia interact with the family's young daughters, and I began daydreaming about becoming a parent.

Mia was the perfect person to build a family around—caring, patient, and exceptionally gentle.

***

Friday began the same way as Thursday, with Mia spinning through ever more confrontational phases of psychosis. Given that she preferred spending time with Luke, I went into work that morning. Being away from home gave me the flexibility to prepare for the weekend without being overheard.

First, I called Mark to update him on Mia's worsening condition. As Luke had predicted, Mark was eager to help, and he liked the idea of using his parents' house as a makeshift crisis center. But he understood my rationale for keeping her home.

Next, I reached out to my dad. He lived most of the year in Indiana but spent winters in a town ten minutes from us. Fortunately, he had recently driven down for the season.

Luke and I had devised a plan together. Mia had scheduled an appointment with one of the priests for later that night. I didn't like her meeting with anyone when she was psychotic, but I couldn't prevent it. In her hyper-religious state, she was seeking refuge at the church. If I denied her that, she would probably think that I was possessed by Satan again.

Luke would drive Mia to her meeting. During that time, my dad would come to our house to pick up the kids. They would stay at his house overnight and, depending on the situation, maybe longer.

I left work early that afternoon. Walking into the kitchen at home, I saw a paper cup sitting on the counter with all of Mia's midday medications inside—she was over two hours late taking her pills! I felt a sudden jolt of anger mixed with trepidation. Luke knew the importance of keeping her on schedule.

He must have heard me come in, and he emerged from the back hallway. "Patricio," he said, "how was your day, brother?" He was pointing at the medication and flashing me the "quiet" sign with the other hand.

"Fine," I said, giving him a wondering look.

"Yo, things been messed up here this morning," he whispered. "Sorry couldn't call or text, she been with me nonstop."

"Luke, the medication—"

"I know, but bro, she wasn't having it. I couldn't get her to take it," he said, his voice still low.

"She has to take it."

"Dude, I tried. It woulda been a fight. I'm telling you, man, a serious fight."

"Where is she now?"

"She's back there." He pointed to the back room. "Same shit. Good one minute and then on another planet the next. Insane shit, hermano."

"Alright, we have to get her to take the medicine."

"It ain't happening unless we tie her down, bro."

Jamie was due home any moment; I couldn't risk her walking in on that. Instead, I asked Luke to resume his watch and quickly texted Dr. Rojas. Two minutes later, Jamie walked in the front door, excited to be starting the weekend. I tried to hide my anxiety but kept checking my phone. Within fifteen minutes, Dr. Rojas had texted back:

> If she won't take it, hold off and add the
> Zyprexa and Seroquel to tonight's dose
> Skip the midday Ativan
> Update me tonight

I relayed the message to Luke. A short time later, Will returned home from school, too. Given that it was a beautiful late October day, the kids wanted to play outside. Jamie began riding her bike around the cul-de-sac, and Will and I started tossing the football. About twenty minutes later, Luke came out to join us. He caught a pass close to me and said, "She's okay, back in your room now."

An hour later, Mia came out of the house through the garage door. She was talking on the phone and sounded natural. "Great, well, we wanted to let you know we were thinking of you on your birthday," she said. "Here, I'm sure your Uncle Pat will want to say hi, too." She removed the phone from her ear and whispered to me, "It's Bobby."

Bobby was our eleven-year-old nephew, Brad and Jen's son. I was relieved to see Mia looking and sounding so normal, and I considered canceling our plans for the weekend. I grinned at her and grabbed the phone.

Mia smiled warmly back at me for a moment, and then went inside. When the call was over, I hung up and put Mia's phone in my pocket. I didn't think much of it. Luke and Mia had to leave for her meeting in a half hour; I would return the phone to her before then. But ten minutes later, she came storming back into the garage. "Has anyone seen my phone?"

"Oh, yeah, sorry. Here it is." I walked up the driveway to hand it to her.

Mia glowered. "Why do you have my phone, Pat?" she growled.

"We were talking to Bobby," I said, surprised at her hostility. "You're the one who called him."

"What are you talking about?" she demanded.

I realized that the kids were watching. I ushered Mia into the kitchen. "Mia, you called to wish Bobby a happy birthday, and then you brought the phone outside so that I could talk to him."

"Oh right," she said. "That's why *you* had *my* phone in *your* pocket."

"Yes, that's why."

She appeared ready to explode. "Pat, why do you keep stealing my phone?"

"I'm not stealing your phone."

"You keep stealing it!" she yelled. "Just stop it!"

"Mia, why would I steal your phone?"

"You tell me, Pat! You tell me!" she roared. "Why are you doing this to me?"

"I'm not doing anything to you." The right response would have been silence.

"You are doing something—you are stealing my phone, trying to trick me!" she cried. "It's hard enough without you taking my phone!" She glared at me, tears filling her eyes. "I need my phone, Pat!"

"Mia, I am not taking your phone."

"YOU ARE TAKING IT!!" she shrieked. "AND YOU'RE LYING!!" She ran off toward our room.

Calling off our plan was out of the question. Soon, Luke and Mia were pulling out of the driveway, and I was assembling Will and Jamie. I informed them that their grandpa was back in Florida and wanted to see them. He would be picking them up in a half hour to go to the movies, and then they would spend the night at his house. As expected, they were thrilled to see my dad and, I think, relieved to be getting away. I helped them pack an overnight bag, and he arrived right on cue.

With the kids gone, the house was strangely quiet, but my stomach was queasy. Experience told me to double-check the lock on the back door of the lanai, and that started me thinking about the way the last psychotic episode had ended. Soon, I found myself wandering aimlessly around the house, worrying about the weekend.

Luke and Mia returned home an hour later. After asking them about the meeting, I said as nonchalantly as possible, "Oh, hey, my dad is back in town. He and the kids decided to go to the movies, so they're just going to stay at his place tonight."

Perhaps I didn't sound as casual as I hoped, or maybe it was Mia's paranoid condition, but the comment didn't sit well. "What?" she asked. "No, that's not right."

"Yeah, it's fine." I tried to sound calm. "The kids were really excited."

"I don't want them to spend the night at your dad's. I'm not comfortable with that."

"They've done it before." This was technically true, although it wasn't common. He usually stayed at our place.

"No, the kids need to be home with us tonight! I don't like it at all. What if your dad hurts them?"

"Hurts them?" I asked incredulously. "What are you talking about? My dad loves the kids, and they love him. He would never hurt them."

"You don't know that!"

"I do know that."

"He could hurt them. He could molest them!"

"Molest them? Mia, how can you say that?"

"Things like that happen all the time, Pat!" she claimed. "This is our kids we're talking about."

"Yeah, and it's my dad we're talking about." I was getting offended in spite of myself. "Mia, the kids will be fine."

"I should have just as much say in this as you! They are my kids, too!"

"Yes, they are," I agreed, "but tonight you weren't home, and I made a decision. The kids are at the movies with their grandpa, and that's a normal thing. I'm sorry, but that's the way it is."

She scowled and rushed to our guest room, slamming the door and yelling, "I'M JUST AS MUCH THEIR PARENT AS YOU ARE!" Luke was standing in the kitchen, having witnessed the whole thing. He shook his head when I looked over at him.

"That went well," I said. "An auspicious beginning to our night."

"Could have been worse," he replied. "At least you got the kids out. Now it's you and me, hermano."

The next hour was uneventful. Mia remained holed up in the guest room, and Luke disappeared to the back of the house. Silent and alone, I started making dinner. Once it was ready, Luke and I tried to persuade Mia to join us at the table.

"Babe, please come out and eat. You must be starving," I pleaded.

"I'm not eating with you, Pat. Just go away!"

Luke rolled his eyes.

"You have to eat," I said.

"I don't have to do anything," she whimpered, her mood shifting quickly. "I can't believe you don't support me—not with the kids, not with the treatment center, not with anything." We heard her begin to cry.

"Yo, whatever, Mia," said Luke. "When you get hungry, come on out. I'm gonna eat."

"Mia, babe, I love you, and I'd really like to eat dinner with you." I sighed, my head against the door, but she didn't respond.

The guest room was located at the front of the house. I noticed that the front door was unlocked, so I quietly walked forward and turned the bolt. Then, after five minutes of listening miserably to Mia's muffled sobs, I joined Luke for dinner.

After we had eaten and cleaned up, Luke and I made our way back to the guest room. With nothing else to do, we sat on the floor next to the door. It was slightly after 8:30 p.m., and we could see the dark sky through the front windows of our foyer.

After twenty minutes, the door opened. Mia walked out, calm and collected, and sat down on the floor next to us. "What the hell am I doing in there?" she asked. I looked blankly at Luke, who glanced from me to Mia.

"It's cool," he said. "Sometimes I need time to myself, too."

"No, this doesn't make any sense," she said. "I don't even know why I'm in there."

Neither Luke nor I dared bring up the kids, so we let her comment sit in the air. Mia rubbed her eyes. "What is happening to me? Why am I acting like this?"

Again, Luke and I let the moment linger. "Are you hungry at all, babe?" I asked finally.

"No, I'm not hungry."

The three of us sat in awkward silence for a few more minutes. It was a strange scene. The glow from the outside streetlamp spilled through the windows, but otherwise we were sitting in darkness.

"Thanks for being here, you guys," she said, "and for putting up with me."

I marveled at the bizarre swings in her clarity and disposition. The highs and lows were exhausting.

"Wouldn't want to be anywhere else but with you," I responded, almost tearing up.

As comforting as it was to hear her sound lucid, I couldn't relax. First, I was apprehensive about the next down cycle; by this point, I knew it was coming. And second, she hadn't taken her pills that day. She was due for her nighttime dose, but I had no idea how to broach the subject.

"Pat," she said abruptly, rotating to face me, "I know I need to take my medication. I'll take it, okay, just give me a little more time?"

I sat looking at her, startled by the question. It was hard to believe she was seeing the situation from my perspective, let alone that she had remembered the pills. "Yeah," I said, "okay."

We sat talking for a while, the three of us. Most of the time, Luke and Mia reminisced about events from their childhood. Someone listening to the conversation wouldn't have noticed anything odd. The room grew darker and darker.

After about forty-five minutes, Mia stood up. "I gotta check my email," she said. "I'll be in the study."

"Okay," I said, standing up with her, "I'll get your medication together." Mia didn't respond; she spun around and walked away. I turned to Luke, eyebrows raised in question.

"Don't worry, bro," he said. "She agreed to take it."

"Right, but does she even remember that?"

Five minutes later, I had her medication in a paper cup and was standing at the door of the study, a glass of water in my other hand. Mia was scrolling through her messages on the computer.

"Here you go, babe," I said. "Time to take your medication."

"I'll take it, just not now."

"I think it's time to take it," I replied firmly. It was already past the designated hour for her evening dose.

"No, it isn't time to take it," she said slowly, treating me like a child. "I'll tell you when it is time to take it."

"Mia, I—"

"Jesus Christ, Pat!" she cried. "Not now, I said!"

I backed away, unsure what to do. Retreating to the kitchen, I put the medication on the counter. Then I thought better of it, remembering what Alex had said. Hustling back to our bedroom, I unlocked the safe and stashed the cup inside. Then I texted Dr. Rojas:

Mia refusing to take the medication

He responded immediately:

> She has to take it
> No choice

I sat on our bed, staring down at his text. I began weighing the options. I could try again, hoping that Mia would change her mind. I could reason with her or try to bribe her. Neither of those seemed promising. Luke and I could hold her down and force her to take the medication, but how do you force someone to swallow a handful of pills? My heart was pounding; the seconds crept by.

After about twenty minutes, I walked slowly back to the study. Gathering my courage, I stepped into the doorway. Mia looked up from the computer screen. "It's a quarter to ten, Mia," I said, "and it's time to take your medication."

"God, you're something," she sneered. "You want to keep me medicated so that you can control the kids, is that it?"

I didn't respond.

"Drug me up, Pat?" she cried. "Keep me under your control!"

I stood staring at her.

"How do I know what's in those drugs?" she yelled. "You could be giving me anything! You and your mind-controlling medication. Why don't you take it, Pat? Why don't you take it!"

I took a deep breath but maintained my poise. "Mia, the medication is for you. I'm not trying to control you; I'm trying to help you. Now, I am going to get your medication, and when I come back, you are going to take it."

I returned quickly to our room. I could hardly open the safe, my hands were shaking so badly. I was scared; I didn't know what we were going to do if we couldn't convince her to take the medication. Grabbing the cupful of medicine, I hurried back to the kitchen for a glass of water.

As I was standing at the sink, I heard the haunting sound of the lanai door clanging. Suddenly, Luke was shouting, "No! No, you don't!"

I ran to the window and saw that he had thrown open the back slider and tackled Mia, who had been trying to escape again. He was now carrying her forcefully back into the house.

I seized the medication, ran down the hallway, and lunged into the back room to find Luke restraining Mia on the floor. He was sitting on her legs and had her arms pinned to the carpet with his hands. They could have been little kids again, wrestling playfully. But they weren't; they were grown adults engaged in battle.

Luke seemed calm, like he had the situation under control. Although he was a thin guy, he still weighed considerably more than his petite sister. Mia was writhing, trying frantically to break free. She looked wild again, like she had in the crisis center—a rabid animal caught in a cage. She was screaming, "You think you can take me, Luke? You think you can fucking take me!"

Then she whipped her head around and caught sight of me, holding the medication. "Think he's going to protect you, Pat?" she leered at me, baring her teeth. "He can't fucking protect you! I'M GOING TO KICK YOUR ASS, PAT!"

Time froze; I was watching the horror movie again. Mia was the most gentle and caring individual I had ever met, but in that moment, if it weren't for Luke, she would have assaulted me.

I found the strength to say, "Mia, you have a choice." My voice was restrained, but the adrenaline was pumping violently through my body. "You can take your medication now, or I will call 911. If I call 911, they will take you back to the crisis center."

I wasn't sure how the thought of resorting to 911 had popped into my head, but instinctively I knew it was the right decision. Luke and I had no way of forcing Mia to take the medication; if she wouldn't take it, the treatment center was the only alternative.

"Do you understand your options?"

Mia looked up at me and spat. "I UNDERSTAND THAT YOU'RE GOING DOWN, PAT!! YOU'RE GOING DOWN!!" She intensified her fight, but Luke didn't look fazed.

I pulled out my phone. "Stop struggling now, Mia, and take the medication, or I call 911."

She was arching her back, pushing madly against Luke's weight. She wasn't about to surrender.

I dialed 911. It was the first time I had ever called the number. Within ten seconds, a woman answered. "This is 911, what is your emergency?"

"My wife is psychotic and won't take her medication," I stammered. The woman asked a few more questions. Within two minutes, we heard sirens approaching from a distance. Suddenly, someone began pounding at the front door.

I ran through the house and, passing through the kitchen, saw red lights reflected in our foyer. Two firefighters were standing on our porch, knocking loudly and peering through the windows.

I unbolted the door, throwing it open. "Sir, we are here for a domestic disturbance," cried one of them; she was dressed in full uniform. She was shouting because the sirens were deafening. A fire truck was parked in our driveway behind her, the lights flashing brightly.

"Yes, come in!" I responded. "It's my wife. She's psychotic and won't take her medication!"

"Where is she now, sir?" the woman asked. They had shut the door, blocking out some of the noise.

"She's in the back room. My brother-in-law is holding her down," I answered, without thinking about how strange it sounded.

The firefighter started walking that way. I began following her, but the other one stopped me. "Sir, I'll need to ask you a few questions." He had sympathetic eyes but a formal demeanor. Glancing behind him, I saw a police car join the fire truck in our driveway.

Things were happening quickly. The fireman had a clipboard and was peppering me with questions. They had to do with Mia, but he was also grilling me, wanting to know if I had been drinking or if there were any drugs in the house. Without grasping his intent, I started talking about Seroquel, Zyprexa, and Ativan.

In the midst of this, the other firefighter brought Mia out of the back room. Luke was nowhere to be seen. I was still answering questions as Mia was escorted past.

"Babe?" I asked. "Are you okay?"

"Sir, please!" snapped the firefighter. "Do not interact with your wife."

She led Mia to our front porch and was met by two police officers. They made Mia sit and began interrogating her, too.

After another couple of minutes, the fireman turned his clipboard around and asked me to sign the form he had completed. I glanced at some kind of report, but it was hard to focus in the confusion. Scribbling my signature across the bottom, I turned to the front door, but the fireman put his hand to my chest.

"Sir, you need to remain inside," he commanded. "We will handle the situation from here." He joined the others gathered around Mia.

I stared out dejectedly at the unfolding scene. Mia was crying, her eyes red and puffy. She was as scared as she had ever been. Uniformed officers surrounded her, with sirens blasting and lights pulsating in the background.

I couldn't hear what they were asking, but I knew her face by heart; I could read her lips in response. She kept answering, "I don't know why he called you. I don't know." Tears began streaming down my face, too.

The policemen kept asking her questions, but Mia couldn't understand what was happening. I watched her say, gulping between sobs, "He must have thought it was something bad, but it wasn't. It was only Kaopectate because I had an upset stomach." She was crying harder now, pleading with them. "It was only Kaopectate."

I had never seen Mia take Kaopectate, but watching her talk about it was torture. All I wanted was to rush out and comfort her, but the situation was out of my control. The officers were standing Mia up, putting her against the wall, and pulling out handcuffs. It was too much; I leapt for the door. As soon as I opened it, the fireman yelled, "Stay in your house, sir! Stay in your house!"

In disbelief, I watched as they cuffed Mia's hands behind her back while she wept uncontrollably. Having pledged my life to this woman, I was now helpless as they forced her into the police car. Even worse: I had called in her persecutors.

A crowd of neighbors gathered on the road, observing in silence. Some stood on our lawn, trying for a closer view.

Suddenly, the fireman was standing in front of me again. "Sir, your wife will be involuntarily committed to the Gulfshore Treatment Center. The police are taking her there now."

Then, as quickly as it had started, the scene ended. The police car pulled out and disappeared around the corner; the fire truck followed immediately behind. Silence and shadows fell across the neighborhood. The gawkers scattered, returning to their homes once the show was over.

But the image of my handcuffed wife remained etched across my vision as I gazed miserably out at the driveway. Not only did I feel that I had failed Mia, but an immense calm was flooding my exhausted body. The house was serene again, and my feeling of relief was mixed with a colossal sense of guilt.

Luke's voice finally broke my trance. "That was some crazy-ass shit."

Turning from the foyer, I found him sitting on the couch in the living room. He didn't look nearly as weary as I felt. I went to the refrigerator, took out two beers, and joined him.

The house was deadly quiet. I handed him a bottle. "Yeah, I don't know what I would have done without you."

Luke nodded.

We sat in silence, slowly draining our beers. I had to face the truth: Mia was not improving. Her illness was becoming increasingly volatile and more violent.

I took a deep breath, holding the air in my lungs and closing my eyes. Was it possible that Mia had a long-term and serious mental illness, one that had altered her personality forever? I had to consider that possibility.

But then I remembered her moment of clarity days before, when we had finally connected through the haze of her disease. The old Mia was still inside, and I knew that if I gave up hope, she might be lost forever.

I imagined her in the back seat of that cop car, barreling across town with the sirens blaring. Soon, she would be imprisoned again in the crisis center, the one place that she most reviled—alone, scared, and confused.

I would not lose faith; I would not stop fighting.

Taking another swig from my bottle, I steadied myself for the next phase of the war.

14.

THE ADVOCATE

School of Fish
"Euphoria"
0:28–1:19

It was sad leaving Texas, but Mia and I were excited to return to Harvard. We had been selected to serve as proctors, meaning that we would live in one of the dormitories in Harvard Yard and be responsible for twenty-five first-year students.

We lived in Mower A entryway for two years, working closely with fifty overachieving teenagers during that time. And we found that when you open your life to that many people and their families, emergencies often occur. We experienced our share of injuries and hospital visits.

But we also learned that mental health problems were the most common afflictions, and some of the most difficult to manage. Given the pressures of Harvard, many of our students struggled with anxiety and depression. These were serious issues and, if not dealt with appropriately, could lead to more complicated situations. Fortunately, we had several resources across campus where we could turn for support.

Even still, the threat of suicide was real. In our short time proctoring, we supported several students coming to terms with the desperate struggles of parents, siblings, or friends. For someone without much experience, the grim consequences of untreated mental illness were eye-opening.

But we never faced a situation where someone became psychotic. The closest we came was through a special relationship with one of our students, David. He was quiet and could be introverted, but his reserved personality hid incredible fortitude. Growing up, his family had been torn apart by mental illness.

When David was little, his mother began suffering extreme psychosis, including delusions and other thought disorders. His father did everything he could to help, but she slid further and further out of reach. David recounted several stories that were difficult to imagine, and I admired his ability to overcome such a traumatic childhood. But he lived in fear that either he or a sibling might succumb to mental illness over time.

One night, he appeared at our door visibly shaken. His brother, who was at a different college, had gone missing and hadn't been seen in over twenty-four hours. David was convinced that his brother had begun his own slide into madness. The authorities had already been notified, and there was nothing we could do but wait.

At the time, it wasn't possible for me to empathize; I had no understanding of psychosis.

In the end, his brother was found and returned safely. But it was tough on David; he kept fearing that a similar fate might be lurking for him in the future. We did our best to reassure him, but words felt insufficient.

"I can't believe what that kid has been through," I said to Mia after he left.

"Yeah," she replied. "Mental illness is tough. There's so much about the brain that we don't understand."

"Psychosis? That's scary. Can you picture hearing voices or thinking people are after you?"

"No, I can't," admitted Mia. "It's impossible to imagine."

***

Luke was still nursing his beer, but I was already up and pacing. I had pulled out my phone and was frantically texting.

"Yo, who are you texting?" he asked. "The family can wait."

"I'm texting Dr. Martinez. That guy runs the crisis center. Maybe he can update me on Mia."

After she had changed psychiatrists, I had sent Dr. Martinez a handwritten note thanking him for his support. It was a sincere gesture of gratitude; I didn't think we would ever see him again. But now, I was hoping it might buy some goodwill.

Within five minutes, I received a response:

> Oh no, Pat, I'm sorry to hear that
> I will contact the center and update you as
> soon as possible

It was late on a Friday night; again, I was shocked by his quick reply. I messaged back details of the past three weeks, including Dr. Rojas's plan for switching from Seroquel to Zyprexa.

Knowing that Dr. Martinez was involved in the situation eased my mind, but I remained anxious. Luke kept me talking to pass the time. Within a half hour, Dr. Martinez texted again:

> Mia is checked in and settled
> Medications have been given
> By all accounts she is fine, so don't worry

I knew he was sugarcoating it for me, but I felt better. At least Mia had finally taken her pills. I remained concerned that she wouldn't want to see me for days, but she was safe. And I was relieved she was in a place that would ensure she took her prescriptions on a regular basis, which was paramount.

The next morning, I wanted to check on Mia without bothering Dr. Martinez again, so I called the crisis center, leaving a message for the medical team.

About twenty minutes later, my phone rang. "Mr. Dylan, this is Dr. Foster," said a voice. "I am the psychiatrist on duty this morning. Your wife is safe and being cared for. She is still suffering from psychosis, and her mood swings have been dramatic. I gave her Abilify to stabilize things."

"What?" I asked, startled. "I'm sorry, what did you say?"

"I said I gave her Abilify. It's a mood-stabilizing drug. We use it to—"

"No. No, that's not in her protocol."

"I'm sorry?"

"We have her on a strict protocol. Dr. Martinez knows the details."

"Mr. Dylan, Dr. Martinez is not here. In my professional opinion, Mia needed Abilify to stabilize her moo—"

"No, no." I was becoming upset. "The last thing we need is to introduce new drugs into her system. We've had a problem with the Seroquel, potentially caused by her migraine medication, and we are moving her to Zyprexa."

"Are you a psychiatrist, Mr. Dylan?"

"No, but—"

"Then I suggest you let us do our job."

"Are you married to Mia?" I snapped back. "Have you watched her deteriorate from a loving mother to a paranoid psychotic?"

I paused.

"Have you ushered her in and out of emergency rooms and mental health facilities for over a month?"

Another pause.

"Mr. Dylan, you don't need to become upset," he said.

"No, actually, I think I do." And without much thought, I started tearing into the poor guy. "Listen, I've learned enough about these medications to know that psychiatrists are really guessing. And yeah, you each have certain drugs you like. Maybe you've had a patient or two do well on them. Whatever. They become your go-to drugs.

"But you don't really know how or why they work. And you don't know how one interacts with another. Oh sure, you'll check your little drug guide, like it has definitive answers. But it doesn't. And every time you add a drug to the mix, it gets harder and harder to figure out what might be working and what's not.

"You give them something, hope they do better, move on to the next patient. But those of us who live with them and care for them, we're trying to get them back. But can we do that if you're complicating things with new medications? No, we can't!"

I was almost screaming now. Weeks of frustration were boiling over, but I couldn't stop myself.

"Mia hates the crisis center. And yeah, you keep her safe, and I'm thankful for that. But we can keep her safe at home. What we can't do here is make her take her medication. That's why I sent her back to you—so that she would have to take her medication. But what good is it if you're not giving her the medication that SHE IS SUPPOSED TO FUCKING TAKE!?"

It wasn't like me, but I had never been so irate. For all I knew, Abilify would send Mia into a deeper state of psychosis.

In the silence that followed, I wondered if I had been too harsh. *No,* my internal voice said, *this is important. Don't let up. Mia is depending on you.*

"Look, Mr. Dylan," the doctor began again, "I'm sure this hasn't been easy for you or your family. I apologize if giving her Abilify somehow compromised a plan that you and Dr. Martinez had set. I will speak with him when he arrives today."

"Thank you."

"But I want to remind you that I have dedicated my career to helping people like your wife, and I have been doing it for years. I wouldn't give a patient medication if I didn't believe it would help them."

"Fair enough," I said. "I'm sorry to question your intentions, but it is absolutely imperative that my wife only be given Zyprexa, Seroquel, Ativan, and Restoril. That's it. And she should be given those medications only in the doses and at the intervals that have been outlined to Dr. Martinez."

Hanging up, I immediately texted Dr. Martinez. He didn't reply, and I felt uncomfortable bothering him again.

But what would have happened to Mia if someone hadn't been there to fight for her? Would every different doctor on call have given her whatever drug they happened to think she needed? I wondered if that occurred with other patients who moved through the crisis center.

Later that day, I was apprehensive walking into the lobby. Maybe I would meet the guy I had just berated, or maybe Mia would shun me. But the receptionist gave me a sympathetic smile. "Oh, Mr. Dylan," she said, "I was hoping we wouldn't see you again."

Surprisingly, Mia allowed me straight through. She was on one of the couches, appearing sleepy. It must have been the Abilify from earlier that morning; her head kept nodding.

We sat together for a while, but the conversation meant nothing. Half the time, I thought she had fallen asleep. Finally, I suggested that she take a nap. She jerked her head, trying to open her eyes wider, and then agreed. I helped her to the bedroom, tucking her into the mattress on the floor.

On the way back to the lobby, Dr. Martinez stopped me. "Hold on, Pat," he said, coming out of his office. "It's a nice day. Let's take a walk together."

We didn't speak as we passed through the building, but as soon as we stepped outside, I said, "Hopefully, the folks around here weren't too offended by my call this morning."

"It's okay, Pat," he laughed. "Actually, no one was surprised when they heard about it. Mia is lucky to have you.

Psychiatrists will always forgive a spouse who cares so much. We wish we saw more of it."

We continued walking around the parking lot. After a silent pause, I confessed, "She hates it here. I swore I'd never send her back."

"I've spent enough time with Mia to know that's true. But you did the right thing, Pat." He stopped, turning to face me. "I have to be in court next week, to testify. Months ago, a psychotic woman woke up and didn't realize it was her husband beside her in bed. While he was sleeping, she got a baseball bat and beat the hell out of him."

"Jesus!"

"Yeah, terrible. It's not her fault, not really. She doesn't even remember doing it. You don't mess around with psychosis."

"Guess not." I thought of all the time that Mia and I had spent trapped together in our bedroom. "Man, though, I really wish you wouldn't have told me that."

"Sorry, but you have to know the truth about this. No one needs a hero. I'm glad you called 911. It was the right thing to do."

Later that afternoon, my dad brought the kids home. They were in a good mood, having enjoyed time away from the stress of our house. I informed them of their mom's relapse. Neither seemed surprised or troubled.

Their apathy worried me. It was like they were giving up hope, as if Mia would drift in and out of the treatment center indefinitely. But I couldn't think of anything to do about it. Plus, it was probably their best coping mechanism.

I was also finding ways to cope. Lately, I had taken to playing the piano at night. I wasn't a good pianist, but the song "*The Scientist*" by Coldplay had become therapeutic.

The lyrics seemed written specifically for our struggle; the band must have been familiar with mental illness. I began playing it incessantly, finding strength in the knowledge that other people had been through a similar ordeal.

In the same vein, I knew that our former student David had survived something similar. I hadn't spoken with him in years, but I tracked him down. He couldn't believe that Mia was sick; the empathy in his voice was palpable. David had a unique perspective, and I found his insight on managing the kids especially heartening. "Just spend as much time with them as you can," he said, "even if they don't want to talk about it. They need you now more than ever."

Fortunately, that had been my approach. Sunday night was Halloween, and the kids and I had spent weeks planning costumes. Jamie was a fairly ghastly vampire, with a black cape and self-applied makeup. She ran around practicing the line "Good evening, it will be your last," sounding as much like Vincent Price as possible. Will had decided to be a British punk rocker, complete with a London subway T-shirt and Mohawk wig. We had been playing a lot of the Clash for inspiration.

But now that Mia was back in the crisis center, I told the kids that I didn't feel comfortable leaving their mom alone on Halloween night. They quickly agreed; I was proud of them. Luckily, Uncle Luke came to the rescue. He eagerly volunteered to walk the kids and their friends around the neighborhood, donning my karate costume and pretending he knew martial arts.

I was disappointed to miss Halloween, but my visits with Mia hadn't been bad. At least, she wasn't making me wait in the lobby. But she always seemed on the verge of sleep, and spending time with her zombie persona demanded tremendous patience.

On Monday, Dr. Martinez called me at work. "Look, Pat," he said. "I know that you and Dr. Rojas have a plan. And I respect the approach of making a gradual switch. But at this point, in my opinion, Mia is overmedicated. She can hardly keep her eyes open."

As soon as he said it, I knew it was true.

"I think we should stop the Seroquel altogether," he continued. "She's already on plenty of Zyprexa."

"Okay," I said, "but removing the Seroquel abruptly could cause issues."

"I know, but let's do it now, while she's in the crisis center. There's no reason for you to deal with it once she gets out. Plus, her psychosis seems much better, at least when she's not sleeping. At this point, all the medication is just overkill."

He was giving me the chance to make the final decision, and I welcomed it. When our journey with mental illness had begun, I was looking to others for answers. Now, I had the confidence to make important choices. I knew Mia better than anyone, and I had seen how she reacted to these drugs.

"I'll call Dr. Rojas and tell him," I agreed. "If we make the change now, she'll probably get out faster, and she'll be on a much better path once she comes home."

Without the additional Seroquel, Mia slowly gained more energy. She wasn't herself, but at least she could stay awake. No wild mood swings occurred, and her psychosis remained at bay. Instead, the blunted personality reemerged, the one that had appeared at the end of her last stay. It was darkly apathetic and paranoid, but not explosive.

Although I was spending afternoons and evenings at the treatment center, in the mornings I was busy searching for the right therapist for Jamie. If a candidate sounded appropriate on the phone, I would book a thirty-minute consultation to meet in person. It took a while, but Jamie was a tough case. I had to choose carefully.

Meanwhile, without Mia at home, the mood was happy and relaxed. Will and Jamie continued playing the question game with Luke whenever they had a chance. "Uncle Luke, where's the strangest place you've ever slept for the night?"

"Easy," he said, looking up from his food. "Sahara desert."

"Sahara desert?" I choked. "You spent the night in the Sahara?"

"Sí, Patricio, several nights." He reveled being in the spotlight again. "Yo, I was traveling with these Bedouins. You know, the guys with the camels and whatnot?"

"Bedouins!" I spluttered. "You were traveling with Bedouins?"

"Yeah, I was in Tunisia," he said nonchalantly, "and I'd never been to the desert. I wanted to see it, yeah? I asked around and ... *pa pa pa, pe pe pe* ... next thing I know, I'm heading out on the dunes, following these guys with their camels."

He looked around at the mesmerized faces and knew his audience was hooked.

"It was real last-minute, though, and mira, I paid for that. The desert's hot during the day, but at night it turns

hella cold, bro. The Bedouins had their tents, but I was lay-
ing out on that sand, just freezing my ass off."

I had given up trying to control Luke's language. The
kids giggled.

"The cold wasn't the worst, though. Mira, I was starving. If you be near the water, you got food. You be in the
woods or forest or whatnot? Food. But when you're on the
dunes, man, you got nothing."

"Didn't you take food with you?" I asked.

"Nah, no time. I'm used to catching my own food,
yeah? That's the way things meant to be, hermano. That's
why I like the ocean. Always something in the ocean."

He was changing topics, moving away from his desert
memories as quickly as possible.

"Like for instance, a week or so before I came here, I
was out diving. It was getting late, yeah, and I thought I
was gonna go hungry. But then at the last minute I caught
an octopus. Good eats, octopus."

"You ate an octopus?" I asked. "Like, an octopus that
you just caught?"

"*Claro que sí.*"

"You ate it raw?"

"Nah," he laughed. "You can eat them raw, but I prefer
to cook them. You ever put an octopus in the microwave,
Patricio?"

"Why would I put an octopus in the microwave?"

"Yeah, probably not." He shook his head at my lack
of worldly experience. "Those suckers pop, bro! Makes a
hell of a racket. Sounds like popcorn going off." He started
making loud popping sounds.

By this time, the kids were laughing hysterically. It was
yet another story that became legend. For weeks, whenever

I asked the kids what they wanted for dinner, they yelled back, "Microwaved octopus!" and started making popping sounds.

On Thursday morning, I was going through the mail at breakfast and found a surprise. It was a card from David, offering me encouragement and a guarantee that Mia's condition would improve with time. He also sent twenty dollars in cash, with the postscript: The money is for the kids. Do me a favor and take them out for ice cream tonight.

I was thinking about David's thoughtfulness on the way to work, when Dr. Martinez called. "Pat," he said, "I'm glad I caught you."

"Thanks for calling. Mia has seemed pretty good lately, at least as far as the psychosis goes."

"I agree. In fact, it's time that she come home."

"Great. We'll all be excited to have her back." But it was a lie; the house was way more tranquil without Mia around.

Less than two hours later, I was walking into Dr. Martinez's office at the crisis center. Mia was already sitting in front of his desk. She looked more tired than she had the previous day, but it was still early.

"Pat, we've been talking about Mia's recovery plan," said Dr. Martinez.

"Okay," I replied, waiting expectantly.

"You have the details of her medication?" he asked, and I nodded. "Let's make certain she takes it exactly how it has been prescribed."

"Right." I reached out to take Mia's hand. She didn't seem that interested, but she didn't recoil, either.

"Also," he said, "I've told Mia that I would recommend therapy for her. Not right away, but as she feels stronger. Her stays here have been traumatic. She should talk through the experience with someone qualified to help."

"I'll make sure we do that." I glanced at Mia. She wasn't registering much of the conversation. "I believe Dr. Rojas works closely with a trained psychologist."

"Good, good." He looked at Mia. "Please try to relax when you get home. Take it easy, and don't put yourself in any stressful situations, okay?"

She nodded, eyelids drooping.

"I don't want to see you back in here again," he joked, but Mia didn't catch the humor. "So, take your medications and get plenty of sleep. If you have trouble sleeping, or start to feel that people are after you, tell Pat."

After the obligatory paperwork, Mia and I drove home in silence. This time the quiet was more familiar, and that made it more depressing.

Once in the house, Mia withdrew to our bedroom for the rest of the day. The kids came home, and I told them that she was back, but there wasn't any interaction. I thought about the first time she had come home, how I had forced the family to spend time together. It hadn't been successful then, and we had another month behind us, a month filled with nothing but strange behavior, sour moods, and detachment.

Making dinner, I thought about the challenges ahead. First, we had to figure out what was going on with Mia. Second, I had to make sure the kids dealt with the stress of our lives in a healthy way, without letting it affect their development. And finally, once Mia recovered, we had to reclaim the intimacy of our family.

Mia joined us for dinner that night. That meant no stories from Uncle Luke, no talking about the school day, and no laughing. We suffered through an uncomfortable silence, the kids with their heads down and me desperately attempting small talk. Things loosened up after Mia sulked back to the bedroom, and then I surprised the kids with a trip for ice cream, David's gift.

After turning up the music in the car, my mind wandered. When Mia and I had started out, we dreamed of building a loving family together. We wanted to form positive relationships with our kids that were based on mutual trust and admiration. But her illness was threatening that dream. The kids were drifting further away from her while at the same time deepening their dependence on me. Nothing about the situation was good.

Shaking my head, I refocused on the sound of the music and Jamie singing along to it. I had no idea what the future held, so I had to set short-term goals.

Keep Mia out of the crisis center, I thought. *If you can just do that, maybe the rest will fall into place.*

15.

THE NEW NORMAL

Big Head Todd and the Monsters
"Dinner with Ivan"
0:44–1:04

Many of my peers at Harvard Business School wanted to become billion-dollar CEOs, or advisers to them, and others wanted to be financial tycoons. But the thought of spending the next thirty years on Wall Street or climbing the power structure of a big company made me nauseous.

Unfortunately, for someone still paying college loans, a lack of enthusiasm didn't justify rejecting potentially lucrative paths. In addition, Mia and I wanted children, so supporting a family was a primary concern. I certainly wasn't looking for sympathy—most people would have loved to be in my position—but the internal conflict was unsettling.

While glancing through course options, I stumbled across a class called *Self-Assessment and Career Development*. The summary read like a self-help book, something about "determining what's important in your life and finding a path that will bring you true happiness."

I had never heard of the professor and was skeptical, but I mentioned it to Mia.

"Are you kidding me?" she replied. "Of course, you should take that class."

"I'm not sure. I only have a few slots, and it would mean I'd have to forfeit *Investment Management* or *Incentive Structures.*"

"What are you talking about? That stuff doesn't matter when it comes to your career. Take the class. End of story."

I listened to her, and it forever changed my life. As part of the course, we completed several personality and behavioral tests. We also answered a number of priority questionnaires. We would be asked countless times and in different ways to rank various aspects of our lives—wealth, health, marriage, family, influence, free time, et cetera. After doing dozens of these, it became obvious what mattered most.

Health was my first priority. Without health, as I had found with Crohn's disease, other parts of life became harder for me to enjoy. After that, the most important things to me were marriage and family. In fact, wealth and prestige, and the other trappings of a business magnate, weren't anywhere near the top. Suddenly, those high-paying jobs that demanded constant time away from home lost their allure.

One of my college roommates, Sam, had started a software company and wanted me to join him. He made a compelling offer, but there was a catch: I'd have to leave business school early. It was the late 1990s, and things were moving at internet speed. For my classmates, the idea of abandoning the MBA program four months before graduation would have been unthinkable. For me, it sounded like a fun way to try working at a startup. And Harvard would let me finish my degree so long as I did so within five years.

Mia didn't hesitate. "If you want to go work with Sam, do it."

"Really?" I asked. "I'd be taking a pay cut from what I was making before business school. If the stock does well, that'd be one thing. Otherwise, it could be a huge waste of time."

"So what if you don't make a lot of money? We don't need it to be happy. What we need is for you to wake up every morning excited about your day."

I was so thrilled at the thought of joining Sam, and so grateful to Mia for supporting me, that I made an impromptu vow. "Tell you what," I said, "if this startup is in any way successful, we'll take a shot at living in Florida. I promise you."

"Deal. I'd bet on you any day, Pat. I'll look forward to our move."

Many spouses would have been upset if their partners had dropped out early or spurned lucrative job offers. But Mia never complained; instead, she guided me to exactly the right decision.

Her support for me never wavered.

***

Although I was relieved to have Mia home, a sense of gloom descended over the house. Moody and snappish, she kept to herself. We tried to avoid her anyway, apprehensive about setting her off.

One of my first priorities was to get Mia in front of Dr. Rojas again. He was eager to see her, and I was desperate to prevent any more bouts of psychosis.

"So, how is *Mia* today?" he asked when we sat down.

"Why do you always ask me that?" she snarled. "Why don't you say 'How are you doing today?' like a normal person?"

Dr. Rojas sat looking at her, smiling pleasantly.

"Did you hear me? I don't like when you ask me that," Mia spat. She continued in a mocking voice, "*How is Mia today?*"

"Would you like me to greet you in a different way?"

"Yes, I would."

"Okay, we'll try this again. Mia, how are you doing today?" he asked. Mia gave short answers to his questions, remaining surly and brusque. She still had paranoid thoughts, and she admitted them, but she wasn't psychotic.

Near the end of the appointment, Dr. Rojas turned to me. "Do you have enough of everything but Zyprexa?"

"Yes, that's right."

"Good. Now, would you like me to write the script for Zyprexa or the generic form?" he asked.

"I don't know." We had been using his samples before the crisis center. "What do you think?"

"The brand-name version is expensive," Dr. Rojas said, "and your insurance probably won't cover it."

"Is there a difference in the medication itself? We finally have things under control, and I don't like the idea of switching." Even slight changes, I feared, had the potential for serious repercussions.

"There shouldn't be, but I can't guarantee it."

"Then let's stick with what's working," I told him.

I went to pick up the prescription later that night. When I gave Mia's name and birth date, the pharmacist looked up at me uneasily.

"Sir, are you sure you don't want the generic form of this?" she asked.

I expected to pay more than usual. "Yes, I'm sure."

"Okay." She started ringing it up. I knew Dr. Rojas had written a script that would last about ten days. "Your total is $1,053.68."

"Um . . . I'm sorry, what?" I asked, trying to digest it.

"It's $1,053.68," she repeated. "There is a generic form."

"Uh, no, that's okay," I said, forcing myself to speak through the shock. As I handed over my credit card, my mind started racing through the math. At $3,000 a month, this wasn't tenable, but I couldn't risk anything that might send Mia back to the crisis center.

I decided to discuss the generic with Dr. Rojas later. And I threw the receipt away inside the store. If Mia had seen the price tag, she never would have taken it.

As the days passed, the family continued to tiptoe around Mia. When she wasn't present, life proceeded on a semi-normal basis. The kids were kids, with homework and their outside activities. And I played the role of single parent: making dinners, fixing school lunches, and trying to keep track of their many appointments and responsibilities.

But when Mia was near, the mood changed. We became quiet, worried about saying the wrong thing. And our altered behavior didn't help the situation; Mia remained highly perceptive. She could sense the abrupt change whenever she joined a conversation. It made her feel as though we were excluding her, and that only exacerbated the resentment.

We couldn't recapture the joy that had defined our family interactions before the illness. I knew the medications were to blame, but it was hard not to take her dour attitude personally. Dinner conversations were especially difficult to manage. Will, older and more reserved, was relatively easy. He mostly watched in silent acceptance. Jamie, on the other hand, couldn't contain herself.

One night, Jamie shared with the family a new theory she was developing. "I figured out something today," she declared. "Vampires are real."

Sudden silence. I looked from Jamie to Mia, whose startled eyes and gaping mouth were frozen in terror.

"That's great, babe." I put my hand on Jamie's shoulder. "But you know that vampires are just make-believe. It's fun to pretend that they might be real, but we know they aren't."

This threw Jamie off, because normally I would have answered with something like, *Oh, is that right? Why don't you tell us the steps in your thinking that led to that conclusion?* She gave me a puzzled expression, but then charged on with her dissertation.

"Well, really, we have no way of knowing that they're not real. Because what are they going to do, tell us they're vampires? Of course not. And if someone gets bit, they become a vampire, so they're not going to tell us, either!"

An uncomfortable pause as Jamie waited for feedback.

"And how are we to know that they're staying up all night? We're sleeping, so we wouldn't know."

She waited again. This was the part where we would throw out contradictory evidence, debating in a light-hearted way the case for and against vampires.

But Mia was now staring at me with a look of absolute horror. As far as she was concerned, Jamie actually believed that vampires were living among us.

I shut the conversation down at that point. Nevertheless, I still had to spend a half hour before bed persuading Mia that Jamie didn't need to see a psychiatrist immediately.

But I finally did have Jamie seeing a counselor, a therapist named Maureen Jenkins. She had a PhD in psychology and considerable experience working with adolescents. Overall, I thought the match was a good one, and I was hopeful that Jamie might open up over time.

Their first meeting didn't amount to much. I escorted Jamie to Dr. Jenkins's office, which included a small table where two people could sit together. After a ten-minute introduction, I left them alone. I knew that Dr. Jenkins's plan was to have Jamie do art as part of her therapy, and it seemed like a great approach. Afterward in the car, Jamie didn't want to talk about it, but I took heart in the fact that she finally had professional support.

With all of the activities and therapist meetings, Luke and I were basically running a taxi service. Mia hadn't been home for long before the fight for control of her car keys reignited. She remained livid that her independence had been curtailed. Plus, she wanted to start contributing again with the kids, and no one could fault her for that.

I discussed it with Dr. Rojas. He advised me that although the Zyprexa blunted her personality, it wouldn't prevent her from safely operating a vehicle. The real culprit was the Ativan, but we had already cut that dose in half, and our plan was to cut it in half again within a few weeks.

Given that Dr. Rojas wasn't overly concerned, the decision came down to trust. For six weeks, I had known where Mia was every moment of every day. The idea of letting her drive off, potentially alone or with the kids in tow, made me nervous. In her current condition, I knew things would be fine; but, as I had seen too many times, her mental state could deteriorate quickly.

I did have one advantage. When it came to technology, Mia wasn't the most sophisticated user. And she took her iPhone everywhere. I secretly enabled *Find my iPhone* on her cell. It made me feel disingenuous, but it also provided tremendous comfort.

As for Luke, he continued to entertain. At some point, I asked him to take Will to a Saturday-morning golf lesson. Luke wasn't a golfer, and the club had strict rules on etiquette. Before they left, I pulled Will aside. "Try to keep him in line," I begged.

They arrived home hours later, and I asked Will how it went.

"Oh, it was fine," he replied, a grin spreading across his face. "The last green got a little dicey, though. I had to plead with Uncle Luke to keep his shirt on."

"Oh jeez," I said, rolling my eyes. "Can you imagine if people would have seen him walking around the course without a shirt?"

"Yeah, well, he didn't take his shirt off, but I thought I better get him out of there when he started climbing the palm trees."

"Are you serious?" I exclaimed. "Those trees are like twenty feet high!"

"I know," he snickered. "Uncle Luke shimmied up easily, like a monkey or something. He wanted fresh coconut."

This wasn't the only story that emerged from that
month. In mid-November, a big fight with Manny Pacquiao
was taking place. Luke found a bar that was showing the
fight, borrowed our car, and drove off after dinner; I didn't
wait up.

Mia woke early the next morning. I heard her rise and
walk to the kitchen. Two minutes later, she came back into
the bedroom.

"Luke is dead," she announced without emotion.

"What?" I sat bolt upright. "What do you mean, 'Luke
is dead'?"

"There's blood all over the porch, and I just checked on
him. He's not breathing." She was reciting facts, with no
trace of distress in her voice.

Immediately, I suspected that she was suffering
another delusion. "Mia, I'm sure Luke isn't dead," I said
with as much confidence as possible. As I stood to throw
on a T-shirt and shorts, I mentally started reviewing the
medications she had taken the night before.

"Yes, he is," said Mia matter-of-factly. She shuffled into
the bathroom to wash up; Luke's demise didn't seem to be
bothering her much.

Walking into the foyer, I scanned the porch and
noticed drops of blood on the tile. I went out to inspect the
scene. Sure enough, I saw evidence of an open wound of
some type; blood was splashed everywhere. Red droplets
led down the sidewalk and onto the driveway, where they
disappeared.

I strode quickly to the back room and looked in on Luke. He was sprawled on the floor and didn't appear to be moving. My heart skipped a beat.

I leaned down to examine him. His face looked fine; I saw no bruises or cuts. Stooping lower, I put my ear to his mouth and could hear faint breathing. *At least he isn't dead,* I thought. And then I realized how ridiculous it was. Dealing with Mia's illness over the past six weeks had me fearing the worst.

I shook his shoulder. "Luke," I whispered. "Hey, Cubano. Get up."

His blue eyes opened slowly. "Patricio? Everything okay?"

"That's what I was going to ask you."

"Yeah, aces, *amigo.*" He smiled groggily.

"Then why is there blood all over the porch?"

"Oh shit," he said, more energy entering his face. "I thought I cleaned that up."

"Mia saw it just now. She's convinced you're dead."

"Ah, damn," he groaned, clearly upset with himself. "Sorry, man, I thought I got it all, but it was pretty dark."

"Luke," I asked in a steady voice, incredulous that he hadn't yet clarified the situation, "whose blood is it?"

"Mira, I was driving home after the fight, and I hit a rabbit."

"That would explain why there might be blood on the car, but there's blood all over the porch."

"I wasn't going to leave that rabbit on the road. That's good eats, bro."

I closed my eyes in disbelief.

"But I didn't skin it in the house," he continued. "That would have really made a mess, yeah?"

"You skinned a rabbit on our porch?"

"Deboned it, too. But like I said, I thought I cleaned it all up."

"You didn't."

"Sorry, man." I could hear the remorse in his voice.

"Luke, where is what's left of the rabbit?"

"It's in the fridge, Patricio. I figured I'd make us rabbit stew tonight," he said proudly, smiling.

No one in the family would want rabbit stew. Jamie loved the little bunnies in our neighborhood and never would have forgiven her uncle, and Will would have been grossed out, too. Mia probably wouldn't have minded, but she wouldn't have eaten it, either.

However, Mia's eating habits weren't what they used to be. She was consuming fried chicken by the bucket, along with loads of bread, chocolate, and candy. She could sit down with us for dinner, partaking heavily of Cuban food, and then a half hour later I'd find her secretly raiding the kids' Halloween candy by the handful.

This behavior was anathema to the Mia I had known. Together, we had prioritized our health, not only with diet but with exercise. Our first date had been a four-mile run together. But Mia had discontinued all forms of exercise, too. I knew it was the medication. Still, it didn't make it easier to witness such a drastic change.

Mia had been petite—five feet two and weighing no more than 110 pounds. But after weeks on antipsychotics, she had started gaining weight. After she had come home from the crisis center for the second time, the bulk accumulated even faster. By mid-November, she had added at least twenty pounds to her frame, probably more. And it came on so fast that it mostly affected her belly.

I knew better than to mention anything about it, but it led to awkward conversations. Periodically, someone would come up to her and exclaim happily, "I didn't know you were expecting!"

"I'm not," she would reply, devoid of emotion and without further explanation.

"Oh, I'm sorry," the person would respond uncomfortably, their embarrassment painful.

With her changing appearance, Mia was moving further away from the person that she had been. She had gone from being caring and kind to selfish and mean, from fun and happy to gloomy and sad. Someone who had been a role model for healthy living was now confusing the kids with terrible dietary choices. It was hard to accept, but it was our new normal, and we each had to deal with it in our own way.

I dealt with it by doubling down on finding the cause of her illness. All of my free time was consumed with research, which included reading everything from scientific papers to random blog articles. Her brother Mark did the same, and we regularly compared notes, but we didn't uncover anything.

As Thanksgiving approached, I began dreading the holiday. The worst times at home were the weekends, with the kids around all day and Mia poisoning the mood. Thanksgiving would be an extended weekend, and we would be adding more people to the mix. I didn't know how Mia would respond, but I knew she would be especially upset if we skipped it altogether. I made plans for us to spend the holiday with my parents and the weekend with Mia's family.

My brother, Brad, and his wife, Jen, along with their boys, would be at my mom's place. I was worried that so many people in a small house would stress Mia's limited patience. I warned the adults, sending an email describing her demeanor and preparing them for potential problems.

Issues began to surface during our drive across the state. Luke was traveling separately, and the kids probably wished they had gone with him. Mia was in a particularly sour disposition. She insisted that I drive, choosing instead to sulk in the passenger seat. But she also demanded that I take a relatively new route. This was before driving apps, and I wasn't entirely sure of the directions.

"This is the exit to 95 that I want, correct?" I asked Mia after two hours, knowing that if we missed our turn, we would have to drive a half hour out of our way.

Silence.

"Mia," I repeated, certain that she had heard me the first time, "is this the correct exit?"

No answer. The exit was approaching fast.

"Mia, it'd be great if you could answer." I wondered what to do if she didn't.

More silence.

"Mia—"

"I don't know, Pat," she grumbled. "Why don't you figure it out."

I tried to stay calm. "Mia, you know this route, and I'd like to make sure we don't go out of our way."

Nothing. I had about five seconds to make a decision.

"Mia!" I cried. "Should I get off here?"

"GET OFF WHEREVER YOU WANT!" she yelled back.

I was so mad, but the kids were glued to my reaction. I took a deep breath, put on my blinker, and swerved into the exit lane. It turned out to be the right call, but it was an ominous start to our holiday.

Once we made it to my mom's place, Mia's conduct became more restrained. She was putting on an act, but everyone could sense her tension. She mostly kept to herself, quiet and aloof. When she had to interact, she was anxious and impatient.

"She seems like she's on the verge of snapping," said Brad the next morning, when we were out running together. "Jen and I are nervous about it."

"Welcome to my world," I said. "Sometimes she does snap."

"Can you and the kids continue living like this? It's been almost two months. It doesn't seem healthy."

"I'm sure it's not, but we don't have much choice."

"You do have a choice."

I knew where he was going. For the past couple of weeks, I had been exploring inpatient programs. They were centers that offered psychiatric and psychological help along with support groups and disease-management programs. "I've looked into treatment facilities, Brad, but I don't think they're an option."

"Why not?"

"First off, they are completely voluntary. Mia would have to choose to go, and I can't see her doing that. And second, they cost a fortune. We're talking, like, two grand a day or more, and most of them have mandatory thirty-day stays. We don't have that kind of money."

"Jeez, really? I didn't know they were that pricey," said Brad. He paused a second. "We'd contribute if it meant Mia got better and you guys could live a normal life again."

"Thanks, I appreciate that, but she's not going to go. She'd never willingly leave the kids for a month."

"Okay, but then what are you going to do?"

"What I have been doing. I'm going to help Mia get better, and I'm going to make sure the kids don't get screwed up because of it."

"Pat," he said seriously, and quit running. "You need to start thinking about what happens if she doesn't get better."

I stopped next to him. "I refuse to accept that the Mia I fell in love with is gone."

"Look," he said in a gentle tone, "I don't want to think that, either. But this isn't healthy for you, and it isn't healthy for the kids. You need to take that into account. I'm not saying that you should give up on Mia, but I do think you need to set a date—say, a month from now. If she isn't better by then, you need to give her a choice: get serious treatment or risk losing her family."

"She's not thinking clearly, Brad," I said. "That's not the kind of thing I can say to her. Besides, it doesn't matter. I'm never leaving Mia."

As I said it, I started running again. Brad took the hint, and we ran the rest of the way in silence.

The morning after Thanksgiving, we departed for my in-laws' house. Luke would be meeting us there, as would Mark and Celia, along with their spouses and kids.

Shortly after everyone arrived, I was in the guest room and heard an argument escalating. Mia was castigating Mark's wife about something, a crescendo in her voice. I ran to the kitchen to find Mia shouting, "You're not perfect, Kim! You're no angel!"

Kim looked startled, clearly unprepared for the verbal assault. From experience, I knew the correct response would be nothing. If one remained quiet, Mia's initial lashing might subside quickly.

Instead, Kim tried to reason with her. "I never said I was," she responded evenly.

"You implied it! Like all I need to do is go to church more often. Like I'm not a good Catholic!"

"No, Mia, I did not say that."

"But you meant it!" Mia cried. "You're so preachy! You're not a perfect Catholic, either, Kim!"

By this time, half the kids were gathered around staring at the altercation in horror. They were used to loud relatives, especially at Delgado gatherings. But this was Aunt Mia doing the yelling; she was usually the calmest one.

I had to take control of the situation, but my typical approach with Mia wouldn't work when she was already shouting. Instead of remaining quiet, I did the opposite. "Hey, what are you screaming about?" I bellowed, "KEEP IT DOWN!"

If watching Mia yell was extraordinary, hearing me roar was inconceivable. Everyone turned my way, including Mia, and the room went deathly quiet.

"Kim—" Mia started, but I cut her off.

"I don't care what Kim said! You need to calm down, Mia. You need to calm down now!"

It was a command. Mia looked frightened but defiant. She had never heard me raise my voice to that level in all of our time together.

"Good." I took advantage of the pause. "You will behave yourself, Mia, or we will leave."

A change rippled across her face, a look of cunning. "Yes!" she agreed. "Good idea. Let's leave. I don't want to be here anyway!" She stalked out of the kitchen.

Feeling all eyes on me, I followed in pursuit. "Mia! Mia, come back here."

"No!" she yelled as she marched into the guest room and picked up her luggage. "We're leaving! I'm not staying here!"

Mia's parents had a full Thanksgiving meal prepared, and the kids were excited to spend time with their cousins. I felt guilty at the thought of leaving but knew it was probably for the best. Mia had clearly reached the end of her limited patience.

"Fine," I said, maintaining my confident tone, "I'll tell the kids to get their things packed."

"No. The kids will stay here. Luke can bring them home on Sunday. You and I need time alone to figure things out."

I didn't want to leave the kids. I feared it would be difficult for them, especially Will. The work with his therapist was going well, but he still preferred being close to me. I also wondered what we needed to "figure out." It sounded suspiciously like getting back to "the truth."

"If we leave, the kids leave," I said. "They're staying with us."

"Why don't you ever want to be alone with me?" Mia shouted. "The kids aren't babies, Pat! They'll survive here for two days on their own!"

She was right, of course. The kids would be fine without us; in fact, they'd probably be happier in a normal environment. But it would be hard on me. The kids gave me the strength to deal with the challenges of Mia's illness.

I started to gather my stuff slowly, buying time to think. My first priority was to remove Mia from the situation. With her gone, the family might enjoy a semi-normal holiday, and no more bizarre memories would be created for the cousins.

"Fine," I said sadly, "put your things in the van. I'll meet you out there."

Back in the kitchen, I found people trying to pretend that life was normal. I motioned to Mark to follow me into the other room. "This might be tough on the kids," I said, "but I gotta get Mia out of here."

"Do what you have to do. We'll take care of Will and Jamie."

"Thanks." I went to find Will. He was playing upstairs with his cousins.

"Hey, bud," I said, pulling him aside. "Mom is upset, and it's best if I take her home. But I want you to stay here with the family. Uncle Luke will drive you and Jamie home on Sunday."

"But I want to stay with you," he whimpered. "I've been looking forward to spending time with you."

"I've been looking forward to it, too. But Mom's not doing well, and I have to take care of her."

His pleading eyes started to glisten.

"Hey," I said gently, giving him a hug. "It's only for two days."

"But it's two days that I don't have school."

"I'll make it up to you. Mom needs my attention right now."

"Okay," he mumbled.

"Thanks for understanding." I released him with a fake smile.

Jamie was downstairs, and if she cared that we were leaving, she didn't show it. She was excited to play with her cousins and seemed relieved to have a few days free of tension.

Ten minutes later, Mia and I were back in the minivan. Mia continued to curse Kim under her breath, ignoring me from the passenger seat. It was the worst Thanksgiving in memory, just like it had been the worst Halloween. I wasn't looking forward to Christmas.

Reflecting on the conversation with Brad, I wondered if he had a point. Maybe it would be best for the kids if Mia weren't around. *Maybe it would be better for me, too?* I thought. Her presence reminded me of the way our lives were before her sickness. The sadness and loneliness were crippling. Despair permeated my thinking during most of the drive.

But then, as we neared the end of our trip, I recalled the fear of waiting for Mark to deliver the results of her brain scan in the ER. As bad as things seemed, at least we still had Mia. And that meant that we still had hope.

I put all thought of abandoning her to an inpatient facility out of my mind. I was afraid of the consequences if we didn't keep her close.

Our family seemed to be hanging on by a thread as it was.

16.

THE LONG TITRATION

Indigo Girls
"Love's Recovery"
3:33–4:00

It was a perfect fall day, and Mia and I were walking through Harvard Yard during our second year as proctors. People were enjoying themselves, lounging among the fallen leaves under the tall oak and elm trees. As we strolled along, we passed a father sitting with his two-year-old son. The boy was perched on his dad's lap, leaning back, staring down at a picture book. The father read in an animated voice, arms wrapped around the child, holding him securely.

Suddenly, the incredible desire to become a parent flooded over me. "I want one," I said to Mia.

"Me too," she responded simply.

Will was born ten months later. Jamie came along twenty months after that. Mia and I read every book we could find to prepare ourselves for parenthood. We took the classes and organized our apartment. We picked out names, assembled the crib, and childproofed the kitchen. We thought we were ready.

And then we discovered that nothing can really prepare you. Parenthood is like jumping off a cliff into the ocean without a life jacket. You crash in headfirst, and then you're swamped. If you're lucky, you have a partner who can hold you steady while you recover from the fall.

When I graduated from college, my mom gave me a scrapbook. Alongside the old photos, she had pasted notes that offered advice for life. One read: *I've learned that if your children feel safe, wanted, and loved, you are a successful parent.* That phrase struck a chord, mostly because it captured how I felt growing up. When I became a father, it became my guide.

I turned to it often when I found myself in unfamiliar situations where the right word or action was paramount. *What would my mom do?* I would imagine. *What would she say?* But I didn't have to face it alone; Mia was always by my side.

And then she became sick. And then she became a different person. And then everything that made our family strong and special started to crumble away.

Keep them feeling safe, wanted, and loved, I kept repeating to myself. *Safe, wanted, and loved.*

***

Mia and I spent Thanksgiving weekend together, but we never figured anything out. She insisted that we organize our files, so we spent hours reviewing old insurance policies and tax forms. It was awkward and weird. We did go out to dinner together, our first date since her illness started. But we were like two strangers, sitting mostly in silence. I was glad when Luke returned home with the kids.

By early December, an entire month had elapsed since Mia had been hospitalized. The Zyprexa had stabilized her thought process. Even though the medication wreaked havoc on her personality, I was thankful that we had it. Anything was better than dealing with the psychosis.

About that time, Dr. Rojas and I decided to move to the generic form of Zyprexa, olanzapine. As I was learning, he took a conservative approach to everything. We phased in olanzapine gradually, mixing it with the brand-name version over time. It worked well, and after a few weeks, Mia had fully transitioned from Zyprexa without any issues. It brought the cost of her medication down by over 95 percent.

Mia still took half the dose of Restoril at night, more as a precaution to ensure that her sleeping patterns remained normal. We had cut the Ativan considerably as well, only including a small portion now as a complement to the antipsychotic. Once we lowered the olanzapine dose a few more times, Dr. Rojas was planning to eliminate the Ativan altogether.

The effect of decreasing both the Restoril and Ativan was that Mia's short-term memory improved. It meant fewer fights and suspicious looks. We weren't continually being blamed for things we didn't do, and we weren't being asked the same questions over and over.

She also began contributing around the house again, sharing basic chores like laundry and shopping. In addition, she resumed cooking, which was a godsend. Mia was an excellent chef, and no one missed my mediocre attempts at dinner.

Although she became more active in the house again, she remained somber and unpleasant, mostly keeping to herself. And with Mia either busy or isolated during the day, Luke began to feel superfluous.

"Yo, I need to give her room," he told me one day in mid-December. "She's never gonna feel normal with me hanging around."

"You're probably right," I agreed, but I didn't want him to go. What if Mia turned psychotic again? He sensed my hesitation.

"I'll stay close, Patricio. Mark got some land up in Georgia. I'll go up there and live rustic for a bit, eat deer and fish and whatnot. I been getting too soft here anyway."

I laughed. "Yeah, imagine how weak you'd be if you actually used the bed."

He scoffed, and then turned serious. "It's six or seven hours away. If Mia starts to get trippy, I'm back in a heartbeat, yeah?"

I reluctantly capitulated, and he set a departure date. I wanted to do something for him, given all he had done for us, but I knew he would never accept a gift. The timing was fortuitous, however; he couldn't refuse a Christmas present from the kids.

Knowing his love of electronic gadgetry, the kids and I bought him an iPad and had a blast loading it with wacky, survivalist-type programs. One provided navigational charts for every body of water on the planet. Another was an electronic manual for existing alone in the wild. After inscribing the back with the words *Cubano Perdido*, we enclosed the whole thing in a rugged waterproof case.

On the morning of his departure, Will and Jamie presented Luke with their gift. He was caught off guard and flashed me a wary expression, but once he opened it, he became mesmerized. The kids showed him how to use it, excitedly pointing out all the functionality. But Luke wasn't one for long goodbyes. After twenty minutes and a few hugs, he was out the door.

I followed him to the car he was borrowing from Marcos and Lucia. "Luke, I really don't know how to thank you. We couldn't have survived—I couldn't have survived—"

"No need for that," he said, cutting me off as he secured his spearguns in the trunk. He threw his rucksack next to them. "She seems good now. Let me know if things change."

"I will."

"Family, Patricio." He gave me the familiar bro handshake. "I got nothing but love for you, brother," he added, pulling me into a hug.

After Luke left, we struggled through the holidays in discomfort. Typically, Mia and I would have enjoyed planning for Christmas, figuring out how to make it special for the kids and spending time with family. But Mia wasn't at all engaged, and it was miserable wrapping presents by myself.

By this time, Mia had gone from sleeping barely six hours a night to getting eleven hours or more. It wasn't surprising, given all the medications she was taking, but it made Christmas morning especially challenging. The kids woke me up before 6:00 a.m., happy and excited, but Mia refused to rise. Desperate, I took the kids to the back room and made a big deal of watching Christmas movies. Three hours later, Mia was yet to be seen.

The olanzapine made her self-centered. She didn't seem to care about anyone else, not the kids and certainly not me. It was so strange for us, given that she was previously so loving and affectionate.

I thought back to the few moments of clarity when she was psychotic, when the old Mia had surfaced. *She must be somewhere inside this despondent stranger,* I would tell myself, but my own conflicted emotions started to cloud my thinking.

When a loved one suffers from mental illness, you become trapped. You want to remain positive, believing that they will find their way back to health. But faith becomes a cruel torture, tricking you with false recoveries. Your heart breaks so many times that you build defenses against hope. You become torn between confidence and skepticism, between supporting your loved one and protecting yourself.

I found myself living in the present, trying to survive on a daily basis. Any thought of the future was quickly banished.

We had moved out of the acute phase of Mia's illness, when I was concerned about her safety. Surrendering the car was a first step. I had also stopped trying to control her phone usage, having long since given up hope of keeping her illness a secret. I could still track her location, but I never did. And with Luke's departure, she spent most of her days alone.

However, I remained highly sensitive to any deterioration in her thought process. I had become an expert in looking for signs of early psychosis. But until I could see any indication of a relapse, I forced myself to let Mia live independently again.

We continued to see Dr. Rojas twice a week. We had a memorable meeting with him in mid-January.

"So, how is Mia today?" he asked. Dr. Rojas had continued greeting Mia the same way, even after she yelled at him for it. He confided in me later that he did it on purpose. Once his patients could ignore his peculiar greeting and move on, he knew they had improved significantly.

"I'm good," she said, without any frustration.

"Wonderful." He continued with the regular set of questions. We had heard them dozens of times by now. After several minutes, he moved to broader inquiries about how she was spending her time. Then he sat back in his chair and smiled.

"Okay, here's what I think happened," he said. "Mia's situation at work caused her to begin losing sleep. The lack of sleep increased her anxiety, which led to even more insomnia. Ultimately, this cycle led to her psychotic break in late September.

"Seroquel was not the best medication to treat the psychosis. Whether it was the Seroquel itself or an interaction with another medication, perhaps the migraine drug, the illness wasn't truly managed until we switched to Zyprexa. All that being said, I continue to believe that this was a case of brief reactive psychosis."

I had been hoping for this. After my own exhaustive research, I couldn't find any other diagnosis. "That's great news," I said. "So, does that mean this was a onetime event?"

"That's what I believe, yes."

I waited for Mia to comment. When she didn't, I said, "Good. Where do we go from here?"

"As I told you during your initial visit, the brain is a powerful and sensitive organ. It can withstand a lot, but it takes a long time to recover once broken." He was speaking in his pleasant manner, looking from Mia to me. But then he focused his attention on her. "I know you want to get off the medications as quickly as possible."

She nodded.

"But that would be a mistake. My number one priority is to keep you from suffering another setback."

"Yes," she murmured.

"So, we will titrate the medication very slowly. It might take five months or longer before you are off all the prescriptions, and we will watch things carefully."

"Okay."

"Good." He turned to me. "Pat, it will be imperative to follow my instructions precisely. We will be decreasing doses very slightly. You'll need smaller pills for everything. Sometimes, we'll have to cut tablets in half. In those cases, just do your best at guessing amounts."

"Ah, sure," I replied hesitantly.

"Good," he repeated. "We'll lower doses and then give Mia's body time to acclimate. Every time we make a change, you should expect mood fluctuations. They're common."

"Okay," I said, even more apprehensively.

Dr. Rojas then outlined the first two weeks. Most of the tapering had to do with the olanzapine. We would be lowering the dose by slight amounts and then seeing if and how Mia reacted to the change. If she was okay after five to seven days, we'd lower it again. If she had a negative reaction, we'd stay at that amount longer. If need be, we could always increase the dose to previous levels.

The first challenge came with our insurance. Mia had a couple of weeks' worth of olanzapine, all five-milligram pills. Dr. Rojas wrote a prescription for a lower dose, but when I went to fill it, I discovered that olanzapine was heavily regulated. The pharmacy wouldn't execute a new prescription until the previous one had been completely depleted. I tried having Dr. Rojas call, but he couldn't do anything to persuade them, either. It was impossible for me to obtain pills in smaller amounts.

In the end, Dr. Rojas told me to chop the five-milligram pills into quarters the best I could. It was painstakingly difficult, and I cursed the pharmacy with every cut. But as infuriating as it was, I would soon discover that dealing with our insurance could be even worse.

When Mia was severely sick, I didn't have time to consider the ramifications of my decisions. I was reacting rapidly to abrupt changes in her health. Given that we had paid substantial insurance premiums for years, I assumed that the bills would be covered.

The emergency room visit and hospital stay coordinated by Mark at the outset weren't problematic; I owed a small amount for them. The trouble came with the Gulfshore Treatment Center, which sent me a bill for over $30,000. The insurance company refused to pay any of it.

Shocked, I immediately contacted my insurance agent and spent the next several days on upsetting phone calls. In the end, I learned that although the GTC was the only acute mental health facility in our county, and the only one within a forty-five-minute drive of our house, it wasn't technically considered a "hospital" by our insurance. Therefore, the company refused to cover any expenses incurred there.

It didn't matter that the only "hospital" in the county that offered mental health treatment was strictly voluntary and that Mia never would have stayed. It didn't matter that she was taken to the GTC against her will by the police. Nothing mattered to the insurance company.

I fought for hours on the phone, met with my agent, and wrote letters of protest—all to no avail. With no other choice, I called the GTC to discuss the unpaid bill. After asking for the accounting department, I was connected to a kind-sounding representative. I decided to go with the honest and blunt approach.

"Here's the deal," I said. "My wife was so sick that I didn't have time to research the arcane rules of my insurance company. I was naïve; I thought they'd cover mental illness."

"Yes, I do understand that, sir," the representative replied.

"And now I owe you $30,000. But I can't possibly pay that."

After a pause, he said, "We do have payment plans, sir. We could put you on a financing plan to make the amount more tenable. We have three- and five-year—"

"No," I cut him off. "With all due respect, I know how this works. If my insurance were paying this, they would have negotiated reduced rates. They'd probably be paying a third of the retail cost."

Silence.

"So, that's what I'm going to do. I am going to write you a check for ten grand. I can afford that. I'm going to send it to you this afternoon, right after we hang up. And then we're going to be even on this." I was speaking with authority, hoping it would work. "How does that sound?"

Another pause. I waited patiently with my fingers crossed. "That would be fine, sir. We can agree to that," he said finally.

I hated shortchanging the GTC. The care that Mia had received there was so important, especially the attention that Dr. Martinez had shown us. But I knew the retail price was marked up compared to what the insurance companies paid, and even the $10,000 was a stretch for us. Yet again, I wondered how people with limited resources survived mental illness.

By the end of February, we had been through several changes to the olanzapine levels, and the pattern had become clear. We would lower Mia's dose of the psychotropic drug slightly, perhaps as little as one milligram. The next day, she would become even more irascible than usual, lashing out at the most innocuous comment. This would last for two or three days, and then her mood would revert to a less-extreme irritability. It demanded tremendous patience.

Jamie didn't have it. In the years before her sickness, Mia's relationship with Jamie had become strained. Mia was raised in a strict home, and sometimes she would revert to ordering the kids around. Will would usually obey quickly and then go back to whatever he was doing. But Jamie would instinctively bristle.

With Mia's changed personality, the friction intensified. Mia would say something like, "Jamie, brush your hair." And even if Jamie was thinking of brushing it, she would immediately refuse on principle. Normally, Mia would have provided alternatives or offered incentives. Instead, with her illness, she resorted to more forceful commands, which only caused Jamie to push back harder.

On an almost daily basis, I would come home to find Will alone at the kitchen table doing his homework. Jamie would be in her room, having slammed the door after a fight. Mia would have retreated to our bedroom. They were like two fighters escaping to the corners of the ring before the next round. "It's a battle royale today," Will would mutter. "Best stay clear of it, Dad."

I enlisted Jamie's therapist of several months, Dr. Jenkins, to help manage the situation. I still didn't have much insight into their conversations, but Dr. Jenkins could appreciate the challenge. "Pat, Jamie has the independence of a fifteen-year-old, not a nine-year-old," she told me, "and you'll have to treat her like one."

Together, we negotiated a set of expectations between Mia and Jamie. We created a list of chores that the kids had to complete each week. We included Will in it so that Jamie didn't feel singled out. It didn't matter when the obligations were performed—a limited freedom that was important to Jamie. For example, Mia couldn't insist that she clean her room immediately, but it had to be done by Sunday at 6:00 p.m. each week. It gave Mia the authority she needed as a parent but offered some control to Jamie.

Thankfully, the arrangement calmed the fighting, but it did nothing to repair the relationship. Will's connection with Mia was also strained. Her cantankerous mindset was so upsetting that we would all avoid her; she was a dark shadow brooding around the house and spreading misery.

And while the kids were avoiding their mom, they were clinging more closely than ever to me. I did my best to remain positive, offering a contrast to the melancholy emanating from Mia. But that only made their detachment from her worse. I was the fun-loving dad they had always known. Why would they choose to spend any time with their mom, who was so frighteningly different? It made me feel awful, but I couldn't find a better alternative.

I kept telling the kids that Mia's old personality would return in time, but they were understandably skeptical. It had been almost six months without any improvement. And every week, when we lowered the olanzapine dose, their mom would turn from sour to downright nasty.

My relationship with Mia wasn't any better. We were still meeting with Dr. Rojas on a weekly basis, and Mia had started seeing a psychologist who worked closely with him. I was hopeful that the therapy might improve her disposition, but it didn't. The effect of the pharmaceuticals was overpowering.

It was a torture every time I gave Mia her medication. I would carefully assemble the pills into a paper cup and then wordlessly hand them over to her, like the executioner passing the cup of hemlock to Socrates. I knew that without it she could suffer a relapse, but I also knew that it would prevent the woman I loved from resurfacing. I felt more like a nurse than a husband. My resolve never wavered, but my despondency grew.

As the days droned on, I began to examine my own feelings. Since Mia had become so startlingly sick at the end of September, my emotions had run through their own cycle of changes. With shock, I realized that I had been working through the customary phases of grief.

It was an alarming epiphany. With a jolt of horror, I recognized what I was grieving: the death of our relationship. The intimacy we felt for each other, the powerful foundation upon which Mia and I had constructed our lives, was disappearing. The trust, the affection, the closeness—they were slipping away.

And then, with another shudder of disgust, I grasped that I was moving into the last and final phase of grief:

acceptance. Living day to day, not thinking about the future, I had stopped hoping that our house would once again become a place of laughter and relaxation. I had stopped longing for a few stolen minutes alone with Mia. I had stopped daydreaming about growing old with my beautiful best friend. I was on the verge of accepting the illness as a permanent part of our lives together.

But that wasn't right. Maybe my emotional side required a coping mechanism, but my intellectual side had to acknowledge the facts. Mia had suffered a onetime crisis. My research pointed to that. Dr. Patel's first impression had told him the same. And Dr. Rojas's expert opinion, formed after countless hours of working with Mia, underscored it.

We had a couple more months to go of titration. It would be tough, dealing with the wild swings in her mood, but we'd get through it. The fall was a nightmare; the winter had been hard; but spring should be a time of hope. By summer, when all the medications had been painstakingly eliminated, Mia would come back to us. And by the fall, our family would be whole again.

The illness would be a thing of the past.

17.

THE RELAPSE

Van Morrison
"Listen to the Lion"
0:19–1:01

When I left business school, I expected to be involved in Sam's startup for a year. But eleven months later, we took the company public, and leaving became difficult.

Those were the early days of the internet, when little companies with big ideas could attract huge prices in the stock market. Our venture was valued by investors at several billion dollars. It was ridiculous, really, given that we were a tiny organization and far from profitable.

When I joined, I accepted a low salary in exchange for a small ownership stake in the company. Once the company went public, that small stake became extraordinarily valuable, at least on paper. But given various securities laws, we couldn't sell any stock.

After six months, executives of the company were allowed to sell a small portion of what we held. However, we could sell only on one specific day, and we had to decide how much to sell the night before.

This was right about the time that the internet bubble started to deflate, and public companies like ours began losing value fast. But many people believed the downturn would be temporary. "The stock will rebound," some of my peers at the company kept saying, "and it'd be foolish to sell anything now."

These were some of the smartest people I knew, and their attitude started to cloud my thinking. The night before the deadline, Mia provided a much-needed voice of reason.

"Wait," she said after realizing that I was having doubts. "Let's make one thing clear, Pat: we are selling at this price. And we are selling as much as we possibly can."

A month later, the stock had lost over 99 percent of its value—but the cash from our stock sale was in the bank.

Without Mia, I'm not sure what I would have done. Thankfully, I didn't have to worry about it. We had enough to take a chance on moving to Florida to be close to family.

And we could survive a medical crisis without going bankrupt.

***

Mia took her final dose of olanzapine in May. We had met with Dr. Rojas earlier that week, and he was pleased with her progress. Five months of titration had gone smoothly, without any major setbacks. It was difficult for those of us living with Mia, and it certainly wasn't easy for her, but Dr. Rojas's plan had been a success.

"As much as I like you both," he joked, "I never want to see you again."

Mia and I laughed, but we remained apprehensive. The medication was our first line of defense. Even though it had ransacked our lives, we knew it protected Mia. Plus, she had been on some type of medication for almost eight months. Stripping away everything felt like walking naked into the future.

I could sense Mia's trepidation, so I hid mine. Instead, I focused on the promise of leaving the bad memories of the past behind. By this time, her old personality was starting to return, and we could have an honest discussion again.

"I'm scared," she confided the night she took her last pill. "I don't want to become psychotic again. Ever."

"I don't want you to, either; but you heard Dr. Rojas, this was a onetime event. Besides, if it ever happens again, we'll know how to handle it."

"Pat, I can only imagine how awful this has been for you. But for me it has been . . . I'm not sure how to explain this." She paused. "It's surreal even talking about this, but when I was telling you all that crazy stuff, I really believed it." She shuddered. It was the first time we had discussed her psychotic ideas. "I mean, with the devil and the eyes and all that, *I actually believed it.*"

"Babe, that was the disease believing it. Your brain wasn't working correctly."

"Right, I know, but think about this. What do you trust more than anything in the world?"

I wasn't sure what she was getting at. "Who do I trust more than anything? I trust you."

She shook her head. "Not who—what." She was waiting for me, but I wasn't following her. "I'll tell you. More than anything in the world, you trust your own brain. It's the thing you rely on most."

I thought about it. "Yes, I can see that."

"Okay, now imagine if you couldn't trust your own brain."

"Oh my God, how terrifying," I whispered as the truth of Mia's experience struck me. It was incomprehensible, trying to imagine that voice inside your head lying to you, trying to trick you.

"Exactly. Terrifying. So, I'm going to need your help. I'm going to come to you if I'm having doubts about things. I'm going to be open with you and use you as my sounding board."

"Of course; you know that I'm always here for you, babe."

"I know." She smiled and then became serious again. "But it's going to be weird. I'm going to let you into my craziest thoughts and hope that you don't judge me for it."

"I listened to your craziest thoughts for months, Mia," I said. "I never judged you for it."

From that night on, she came to me for thought confirmation. At the outset, she did so frequently. I always tried to stop what I was doing and provide my undivided attention. She would say things like, "I was at Jamie's school today, and her teacher said that Jamie was a 'real character.' I think she meant that Jamie is unusual, with her vivid imagination and everything, right?"

"Yes," I would answer, "that's what she meant."

"Okay, good, because for a second I thought she might be implying that Jamie thinks she's an actual character from one of her books. But that wouldn't make any sense."

"Correct, that wouldn't make any sense."

We had countless exchanges like this. Mia needed to confirm that she hadn't interpreted comments too literally, or that she hadn't misjudged someone's emotional response to a situation. Texts were especially difficult for her, given that so much could be misunderstood.

The approach worked, and she slowly regained her confidence, one interaction at a time. As the weeks passed, we began to see more of the old Mia. Once she started laughing again, sometime midsummer, I knew that real progress was being made. With her laughter came a thawing of the tension that had gripped our house for months. The kids sensed the change, and Mia's relationship with them began to heal.

At the same time, without the medication, her body reverted to its natural metabolism, and her appetite no longer raged out of control. The weight she had gained came off steadily throughout the summer, and her mood and energy levels increased. She was back to her normal rest schedule, no longer sleeping eleven or more hours at night and taking naps during the day.

When the kids resumed school in the fall, Mia felt strong enough to go back to work. She didn't want to return to clinical practice immediately, believing that starting slowly would be less stressful. She had a standing offer to become an instructor in the PA program of a local university. She could work part-time and increase her hours when she felt ready.

By early November, our lives had returned to normal. The kids, now in seventh and fifth grades, were doing well. Will had long since overcome his separation anxiety, and Jamie and Mia weren't fighting nearly as much. Mia was kind, caring, and cheerful again. From the outside, only those who really knew her could sense the changes that the crisis had imparted. She was a bit more specific with her language, a little slower to laugh, and slightly more anxious overall.

Below the surface, Mia was struggling to accept what had happened, and I was struggling, too. I had gone from feeling like an emergency room doctor to feeling like a nurse to feeling like a therapist. Although the frequency was receding, she continued to come to me for thought confirmation. So I knew that although she could override its initial reaction, her brain suffered lingering effects of the illness.

But it was more than that. My defenses against being hurt remained in place. Prior to the crisis, I had complete faith in Mia and the close connection that we had built. It wasn't her fault, but that faith had been shattered. We still had our relationship, but I had already grieved its demise. I was wrestling with feelings of love and hope, on the one hand, and not wanting to relive such an incredible loss on the other.

I decided that time would heal the bond between us. It was unrealistic to believe that our relationship could mend itself in a few months, but we had our entire lives to rebuild. The long agony was over; with patience and commitment, the closeness we had cherished would reemerge.

And then, in early December, Mia came to me with fear in her voice. "Pat, I didn't sleep well last night," she told me abruptly one morning.

"What do you mean?" I felt like Mark in his clinical mode. "Did you have trouble falling asleep? Did you wake in the middle of the night? Are you worried about something?"

She responded with the precision of an experienced patient. "No, I fell asleep fine. Yes, I woke around 2:30 a.m.

and couldn't fall back to sleep. No, I don't think anything was worrying me."

But she was concerned now. Dr. Rojas believed that a lack of sleep had triggered the last crisis, and Mia knew it.

"I'm sure it's fine, babe," I lied, not wanting to fuel her anxiety. "Try not to worry about it. I'll call Dr. Rojas today to see what he thinks."

"Okay," she said uncertainly.

Dr. Rojas was surprised and disappointed to hear from me again, but he didn't seem alarmed. He told me to give Benadryl at bedtime, an antihistamine known for its soporific effect, and to contact him the next day with an update.

That night, Mia took twenty-five milligrams of Benadryl. I couldn't relax until she was breathing heavily, which happened after about an hour. But when I woke the next morning, she was already up, waiting for me.

"Pat, it happened again," she said nervously. "I was up at 3:00 a.m., and I wasn't tired at all. I've just been lying here since."

"Look," I said as calmly as possible, "Dr. Rojas wasn't overly concerned, and we shouldn't be, either. We're fully on top of the situation. I'll call him this morning."

Once again, Dr. Rojas didn't seem panicked. He instructed me to switch out the Benadryl for Restoril. "She isn't going to want to start on strong medications again," he said, "but it's important that we get her sleeping through the night. The Restoril should ensure a solid night of sleep tonight."

"She'll do anything to prevent a relapse," I assured him.

"Good. Pat, it goes without saying that you should watch for any signs of concrete thinking or centers of reference. Anything that seems out of the ordinary."

"She has been bouncing her thoughts off me. I'll know what she's thinking."

"Bouncing her thoughts off you?"

"Yes. Sometimes she has thoughts that might be a bit paranoid or confused, but she's able to see them as such and overrule them. She checks her conclusions with me."

"Good. Keep me updated. I want to know any changes."

Mia took fifteen milligrams of Restoril before bed that night. After forty-five minutes, she was asleep, but I couldn't relax. Planning for the worst, I snuck out and emailed Luke, putting him on standby. After living off the land in Georgia for a few months, he had gone to Mexico. But we communicated frequently; I knew he would return on a moment's notice.

Mia slept for three and a half hours and then woke around 1:30 a.m., fully energized. I had instructed her to alert me if that happened, which she did at 2:00 a.m.

"I've been lying here for a half hour. I'm not going to fall back to sleep; I know it."

"Yes, you are. You're taking another fifteen milligrams of Restoril right now." I rose to fetch the medication.

"Do you think that's a good idea?"

"I'm sure of it, babe." We had to get her sleeping again.

After taking the medication, Mia slept another three hours. I didn't. I crept over to the safe to check our supply of pills, including olanzapine and Ativan. If the war was coming, we'd be ready. Any thought of rebuilding our relationship was forgotten. I was—once again—completely focused on saving Mia.

The next day, Dr. Rojas was startled that the Restoril hadn't worked as planned. He thoroughly supported my decision to give more in the middle of the night.

"Any thought disorder?" he asked.

"Not that she has shared, and I haven't noticed anything."

"Okay, good. Same thing tonight. Restoril before bed and more if she wakes up. Keep me updated."

When I checked my emails, I saw a response from Luke. "I got your back no matter what, Patricio. I'm in Cabo San Lucas, but there's nothing I can't drop in an instant." It gave me a jolt of courage. *Okay, disease,* I thought, *we're ready for you this time.*

Mia taught on Thursdays, and the kids were already asleep when she arrived home that night. After sneaking in to kiss them good night, she came into our room.

"Pat, I need to ask you something."

She was anxious; I gave her my full attention. "What is it?"

"I was testing the students on their clinical interaction tonight, and I think they were videotaping me. Does that seem right to you?"

That familiar feeling of adrenaline hit instantly.

"Hmm, what do you mean?" I asked nonchalantly. "Was someone there taping the students for the exam and you were involved, too, because you were asking the questions?"

"No, I don't mean that. I mean, I think the school has secret cameras, and they haven't told me. I'm pretty sure they have them embedded in the walls."

I didn't want to startle her. The school might have posted cameras in different places, but the idea that they were hidden in the walls and designed to record her was absurd. She was losing the ability to separate fantasy from reality.

"I wouldn't worry about it. They may have a security system, but they're not watching you or anything."

She put her finger to her chin in that quizzical way that reminded me too much of the early days of her psychosis. "I'm not so sure about that."

I changed the subject and gave her Restoril. Once she fell asleep, I texted Dr. Rojas. It was past 10:00 p.m., so I was surprised when he responded immediately. He was as concerned as I was with her paranoia. We discussed starting olanzapine, but he remained hopeful that a few nights of fuller sleep might resolve the problem.

Mia woke again in the middle of the night, this time with her thoughts racing. She was focused on work, telling me about the various students she had tested. She kept repeating her questions and the answers that were given, all the time wondering if the school had caught it on tape. It was bordering on psychotic, and I was reminded of that first morning of the crisis, when she became fixated on a patient in her pediatric clinic. I was relieved when she fell asleep for the second time that night.

By this point, I had plenty of experience with disjointed ideas and paranoia. It was disheartening but not creepy. However, I was stunned at how quickly her thought process had veered out of control. Less than twenty-four hours earlier, we had been sharing rational conversations; that seemed impossible now. Lying in the dark, I began mentally preparing myself for the upcoming days, before drifting into my own troubled slumber.

Surprisingly, she seemed much better in the morning. After the kids left for school, I went to my office to gather up work to bring home. I texted Dr. Rojas details of our midnight exchange. His concern was growing, and he asked me to keep him constantly informed.

As I was collecting my things, I received a text from Mia:

> A man with a white van is watching me walk Chica

My heart sank as I responded:

> What do you mean, watching you?

I was hoping for a rational response; it didn't come:

> He smiled at me but I don't know him
> I don't think he wanted me to see what he was doing

How does one deal with delusions from afar?

> I'm sure he's just working on the cable or the sprinklers or something

I sat waiting, my pulse increasing.

> No, he's not
> I think he's installing a video camera
> It's where the kids get off the bus
> He wants to record them

I took a deep breath, exhaling slowly. The battle had started.

I'm sure it's fine, babe

I'll come home and we can talk about it

Soon, I was pulling into the driveway. I found Mia in our room. A brief conversation confirmed the worst: she was fully convinced that the utility worker, whom I saw when I drove into the neighborhood, was plotting to kidnap the kids.

Without hearing from Dr. Rojas, I gave Mia two milligrams of Ativan. Before, I would have been hesitant to make such a decision, but over the past year, I had become well versed in these pharmaceuticals. I didn't start the olanzapine; I wanted to confer with Dr. Rojas first.

The Ativan calmed Mia down, and I left her in our bedroom on the pretense of doing work. Instead, I began mobilizing the troops. First, I texted Dr. Rojas. Then I sent an email to Luke, asking him to return as soon as possible. I also sent a group email updating both sides of the family. Finally, I contacted one of our closest friends in town. She could help with the kids.

Jamie came home from school first. She immediately knew that something was wrong, and I went into her room to speak with her alone.

"Remember last year when Mommy got sick?" I asked.

"Yes."

"Well, it's happening again. But her doctor and I, we're really prepared this time. We know exactly what to do to help her. But it's going to take time, so she might be acting a little strange over the next few days."

Jamie lowered her eyes and her shoulders sagged, but she didn't say anything.

"So, I wanted to give you a choice. You can stay home tonight, or you can go have a sleepover with Beth." Beth was our friend's daughter; she and Jamie were good friends.

Jamie sat for a few seconds, then responded, "I really want to be here for Mommy, but I think it will be easier for me at Beth's house."

"That's okay." I nodded. "They'll be over to pick you up in an hour." Then I gave her a hug, holding her a little longer than usual. "Don't worry, Mommy is going to be fine."

Will walked in the door shortly after, and I had a similar conversation with him. Surprisingly, he chose to stay home. "I want to be here for her," he said. "If she's sick and scared, maybe I can help."

I smiled. "I'm sure having you around would be nice for her, but Mom might be acting really strange. I don't want it to upset you."

"I can handle it, Dad. Now that I know she's going to be alright, it isn't as scary as before."

Dr. Rojas texted back later that afternoon:

> I want to nip this in the bud
> Let's hit her hard with the Zyprexa
> 5 mg now, 10 mg more before bed

The thought of putting Mia back on olanzapine, or Zyprexa, as Dr. Rojas always referred to it, was depressing, but I knew there was no other choice.

> Okay, I agree with that approach

His next text arrived before I even hit send:

> Restoril 15 mg before bed
> 15 mg more if she wakes up
> Ativan 2 mg before bed
> Zyprexa 5 mg and Ativan 2 mg when she
> wakes up in the am
> Do you have all the medications you need?

I confirmed that no prescriptions were needed.

> Good, keep me updated
> Don't hesitate to call
> I'm here for you both

With that, Will and I faced the night together with Mia. She wasn't happy taking the olanzapine, but she could sense that something wasn't right; she didn't protest. I made her show me that she had swallowed the pills, then I locked all the medications back in the safe. We were falling too easily into familiar patterns.

I warmed up leftovers, and then we decided to watch a movie together. Will had never seen *Father of the Bride*, with Steve Martin, and I thought he would enjoy it. The three of us sat together on the couch, with Mia in the middle and Will and me on either side, holding her hands. Both of us went out of our way to act normal and calm.

Mia could sense our relaxed nature, and I think it helped. Her thoughts were obviously racing, but she desperately tried to sit still. About twenty minutes into the movie, she started asking about the characters in peculiar ways that made it clear she wasn't following the plot. Will patiently and lovingly answered her questions. Before too long, she stopped talking. It might have been drowsiness from the olanzapine kicking in.

In the end, the night was a nonevent. Mia sat quietly during most of the film while Will laughed nonstop. When it came time for bed, Mia and I went through our old ritual. I passed a paper cup full of pills to her, and she swallowed them without hesitation.

I slept lightly throughout the night, waking often to check on her. Every time I did, she was breathing heavily. She woke around 5:30 a.m., having slept over seven hours. It was an incredible victory. At the outset of the first crisis, it had taken much longer to slow down her brain.

She had no energy and wasn't talkative. Without much interaction, I couldn't ascertain how she was thinking. But she wasn't psychotic, and that was reassuring. I gave her the morning medication and texted Dr. Rojas. He replied quickly:

> Good. At noon, 5 mg Zyprexa and 2 mg
> Ativan
> Keep me updated

Mia kept to herself, and I passed the time sending email updates to the family. I sent Luke a message letting him know that the crisis might have been averted, but he was already on a plane to Miami.

By 10:00 a.m., Mia had climbed back into bed for a nap. I was dumbfounded when I walked in and found her sleeping. I excitedly texted Dr. Rojas, ready to celebrate our victory. He was encouraged but remained adamant: I was to give her the additional medication at noon, even if I had to wake her to do it.

When the time arrived, I begrudgingly roused Mia from a stupor. I began with several small nudges and progressed to more-aggressive shoulder shakes. "Hey, Mia!" I resorted to shouting. "You need to wake up!"

Finally, I was able to pull her into a seated position; she was so drowsy that she couldn't open her eyes. "I know you're tired," I pleaded, "but Dr. Rojas wants you to take these." I held out the paper cup, but she wasn't paying attention.

With much patience and prodding, I managed to give her the pills. She grunted periodically, but she never opened her eyes. She was like someone you might see in a movie who has overdosed on narcotics. It felt like instead of giving her more drugs, I should be pulling out an adrenaline shot. When she finished, I gently guided her head back to the pillow. She fell asleep instantly.

The battle never came. The olanzapine snuffed out any threat of psychosis, and all the medication left Mia blunted, weary, and slow. Luke showed up on Sunday but stayed for only a few days. Although Mia remained more paranoid than usual, she didn't need someone watching over her. She mostly slept anyway.

Unfortunately, the medication caused her sullen disposition to reappear, and she once again isolated herself from the family. Her short-term memory went to hell and her diet fell apart. It was familiar to us now, but it didn't make things easier. In his conservative style, Dr. Rojas wanted to be sure that the episode was fully under control, so he kept Mia on high doses of olanzapine for several weeks. We suffered a second Christmas under the gloom of her grumpy moodiness.

As the new year started, we began another drawn-out titration of medication. The usual pattern returned, with Mia's attitude becoming unpredictable in the days following a change in dose. At her worst, she was mean; at her best, she was detached. In every case, she was far from the person with whom I had fallen in love.

At least, like Will had said, we knew she would recover. That knowledge made her behavior more tolerable, but it also made it easier for us to ignore. *Wait until she comes back* seemed to be the unspoken approach among the three of us. Our family, which had been mending deep wounds so effectively during the fall, was ripped apart again.

I felt an overwhelming sense of sympathy for Mia. Before having kids, we had talked with so much excitement about watching them grow. But she had basically missed the past year and a half of their development. Will was midway through middle school, and Jamie was almost finished with elementary. The old Mia would have been crushed at having missed it, even though the medicated Mia didn't seem to care.

As for our relationship, I avoided considering it. Thankfully, my defenses remained strong during the relapse, and I didn't suffer nearly the sense of personal grief as the first time around. Rather than think of Mia as my wife, I found myself viewing her more as my friend. I couldn't abandon a friend to a life of periodic mental crises, where months and months of strong medications left her unrecognizable, but I didn't know what to do.

Dr. Rojas thought Mia had suffered from a onetime event, but it didn't take a degree in psychiatry to question that diagnosis. As for solutions, we were stuck. We could handle the illness, that much was certain. But could we figure out what was causing it?

Could we find a way to prevent Mia from facing a never-ending battle with psychosis?

18.

DESPERATION

Dire Straits
"Romeo and Juliet"
2:57–3:23

After my experience at Sam's software company, I returned to Harvard to finish my last semester of business school. Since leaving three years prior, Mia and I had become parents twice over. Our little startup had gone public, suffered the ups and downs of the internet, and finally merged with another public company.

Remembering my promise, I suggested to Mia that we try living in Florida after graduation. I knew little about the Sunshine State, but it was important to both of us to be near family.

I talked my way into a role at a small investment firm in Sarasota. The city was close enough to family for visits but far enough that we would have independence. I didn't do any homework when considering the job. I met the owner, interviewed with a few employees, and accepted an offer. Mia and I needed a catalyst to jump-start our move, and the position seemed good enough.

In late July, a moving truck came and hauled away our furniture and carefully packed boxes. Prior to our departure, Mia and I signed a contract to purchase a home in Sarasota. We had enough for a down payment and were committed to spending at least two years in the area. We figured a house would be good for the kids and a decent investment if we wound up staying.

We pulled into our new town in early August, and I had my first day of work the following Monday. The tiny business advised wealthy clients in an emerging area of finance. Within twenty minutes, I had met everyone at the company. They were friendly enough, but I soon discovered that poor decisions were being made by the senior executives. They weren't doing things that were blatantly illegal, but their actions made me extremely uncomfortable.

The discovery startled me. At first, I was upset for not having done more research before taking the job, but then I started thinking about the money we were spending on the house. The more I thought about it, the sillier and more reckless our decision seemed. Boston was filled with friends and opportunities. Apart from family, Florida offered nothing, except a questionable role with strangers that I didn't trust.

At noon, I left the office on the pretext of going to lunch. Instead, I nervously huddled in my car and dialed Mia's cell phone.

"We can't stay here," I said when she answered. "We need to call the moving truck and tell them to turn around. We have to get out of buying that house. Let's put the kids in the car and drive back to Boston."

"What?" she asked, caught completely by surprise.

"I won't go into it, but I can't work with these people," I pleaded. "You wouldn't believe what's going on at this place."

Mia didn't ask clarifying questions; she didn't argue. Instead, she let a few moments pass. Then she said, slowly and steadily, "Listen to me, Pat. You promised me two years." She took another pause. "Figure it out."

It was like a physical slap to the face, and I stared blankly at the parking lot around me. She was right. We didn't move to Florida because of this particular job; we moved for more important reasons. I couldn't let one poor decision sour the rest of our plans.

I learned something vital that day. The struggle is okay; it drives you forward, forces you to find solutions. But you can't give up.

You can never give up.

***

It took over four months to wean Mia off the medications the second time around, and the experience was just as unpleasant as before. We were painfully reminded of the remarkable and demoralizing differences between the healthy Mia and the medicated Mia. In her presence, everyone remained subdued and serious. Even Jamie was learning the routine; she kept her imagination reined in.

We restarted our weekly meetings with Dr. Rojas, having swiftly abandoned the goal of never seeing him again. In March, he broached the subject of Mia's revised prognosis. "I didn't expect this setback," he admitted, "but it doesn't change my initial diagnosis. I still believe this was a onetime event."

I didn't understand it. "Dr. Rojas," I said, with as much decorum as possible, "it wasn't a onetime event. It happened twice."

"Yes, but the second time wouldn't have occurred if the first time hadn't been so damaging." He looked at Mia. "That experience was so traumatic that your brain became more susceptible to it happening again. Something in December must have caused you to become more anxious than normal, and that progressed into a degradation of your sleeping patterns. As you lost sleep, the chemical balance in your brain was interrupted, and that led you back to paranoid delusions."

Mia didn't respond.

"Okay," I said, "but even if that did happen, why did the thought disorder start so quickly? The first time around, she was worried about work for weeks before the psychosis suddenly appeared."

"I don't believe it all broke at once back then. This time around, you were attuned to the signals. You were watching closely, Pat, and Mia wasn't hiding anything. Working together, you were able to catch it quickly. The first time around, you weren't.

"We know that the brain can withstand a lot of pressure before breaking," he continued, "but once that happens, it can take a long time to heal. Mia's brain was still recovering and was vulnerable."

"You're saying that these two episodes were somehow related, that one led to the other?" I asked. "You're looking at this as one drawn-out and connected event?"

"Yes. What I'm saying is that the problem came a year and a half ago. What happened in December was an aftershock."

I was starting to understand his perspective. "Alright, but how do we fend off another aftershock?"

"That is the key question," Dr. Rojas responded. "I'm confident that the longer we can push out any potential future episodes, the less severe they will be and the shorter they will last, if at all."

"So, you don't think this is schizophrenia?" Mia asked, nervously joining the conversation.

"No, I do not think you have schizophrenia," he stressed. "It doesn't fit at all." I could see the tension draining from her body at his answer.

"Okay, how do we push out future episodes?" I asked.

"First, I'd suggest you stop working," he said to Mia. "I know that isn't what you want to hear, but your new job played a role in this. You must have been worried about something, even if you didn't realize it."

"Okay," Mia replied, unable to hide her disappointment.

"It isn't forever, just until we put some time behind us. Second, we should do what we can to minimize your overall anxiety. We can't let it affect your sleep. That's where the trouble starts."

"How do we do that?" I asked.

"Mia needs to find activities that will remove stress from her life. We might also try a small dose of antianxiety medication. We could use it as a prophylactic for a short period of time."

"Fine," Mia said, "whatever we need to do. I don't want this to happen again." Her eyes welled up. "It can't happen again. It's so hard on the kids and on Pat." I put my arm around her, but that only invited more tears.

"It's okay, babe," I said. "We just want you to stay healthy."

Dr. Rojas offered her a box of Kleenex. She pulled a few tissues and began dabbing her eyes. "It's not okay, Pat," she whispered. "I'm losing the kids. I'm losing you. I'm missing out . . ."

I didn't know what to do but pull her closer.

"Mia," Dr. Rojas said, giving her a comforting smile, "you are fortunate to have a supportive family. Your brain will heal itself with time."

By April, the second titration had come to an end. Dr. Rojas gave Mia a few weeks without medication before putting her on a small dose of fluoxetine. It was more commonly known by its brand name, Prozac, an antidepression drug that also had antianxiety properties. Mia wasn't excited about taking more pills, but she was determined to avoid another setback.

We reverted to our previous interactions, with Mia coming to me frequently for thought confirmation. I didn't mind, and as Dr. Rojas had pointed out, the transparency helped us gauge her mental clarity. She was still having issues with paranoia and taking people too literally, but once again she was able to override her initial reactions.

We knew the fluoxetine would take a few weeks to work, and we were both hopeful that it would add another layer of defense. But later that month, it became obvious that this new strategy wasn't viable.

I was pulling into my office parking lot after lunch when I received a distressing text from Mia:

> Something isn't right
> I've never felt so depressed

Her words glowed on the screen before me.

Did something happen this morning?

I waited impatiently for her reply.

No, but this isn't normal
I feel really down
I feel suicidal

I stopped texting and immediately called. She answered quickly. Her day had been okay until a few hours prior, when she had started to feel depressed. It steadily worsened until she felt compelled to alert me. I kept her on the phone until I arrived home.

For two years, we had been fighting mania, but depression had never surfaced. It was the main reason that a diagnosis of bipolar disorder was inappropriate. After discussing it with Dr. Rojas, he firmly believed that the fluoxetine was to blame; suicidal thought was a rare but well-documented side effect. Mia immediately stopped taking it.

Thankfully, once she quit the medication, the depression rapidly subsided, and all thoughts of suicide vanished. I was astonished that a chemical could have such a focused and frightening effect on her brain. Anyone who thinks that mental illness is "all in someone's head" has had no experience with these drugs.

After that scare, we abandoned the part of the plan that involved more medication. Instead, Mia concentrated on finding natural ways to remove anxiety from her life. She started therapy again, and she experimented with biofeedback techniques and meditation.

As the spring moved into summer, it felt like a repeat of the previous year. The old Mia gradually reappeared. Her diet returned to normal, and the additional weight melted off her frame. She gained energy and enthusiasm, rejoining the family and restoring her broken bonds with the kids. Will and Jamie accepted her overtures more readily this time around, the benefit of time and experience giving them a more mature view of the illness.

But for Mia and me, something was different. Before, we thought that the worst was behind us and that she wouldn't suffer again. Now, we knew that the illness remained, lurking in the darkness, and the only way to keep it at bay was sufficient sleep. For that reason, we became hyperaware of Mia's nightly patterns. Our conversations revolved around how many hours she had slept or if she had woken up during the night. I didn't know how she fell asleep at all with the pressure. She became well versed in valerian teas, melatonin, and other natural sleep aids.

By late August, our house had returned to normal yet again, or as normal as possible given our constant vigilance around sleep. The kids were doing well in school, now in eighth and sixth grades, and Mia's personality was fully restored. Our relationship hadn't yet been mended, the intimacy still lacking. It was my fault. My defenses remained high. I wasn't a husband but a clinician, watching my patient with concerned eyes.

Then, in September, Mia woke me in the middle of the night; she couldn't fall back to sleep. As we had planned, she roused me after lying awake for thirty minutes.

"Okay, let's do twenty-five milligrams of Benadryl," I said. "That's what Dr. Rojas would say." She took the pill, and I waited quietly next to her in the dark, until she began twitching. It took over an hour, but at least it worked. We contacted Dr. Rojas in the morning.

> Forget the Benadryl
> Go right to Restoril tonight
> 15 mg and then 15 mg if needed upon waking
> Keep me updated

The pattern was familiar, the results devastating. We fought hard to keep Mia asleep, fought with medication and herbs, meditation and relaxation. Nothing worked. The Restoril kept her asleep for three hours at a time, if we were lucky. She and I both knew what was coming next; it was like watching someone drown in slow motion, but being helpless to throw a lifeline.

Some weeks prior, we had arranged a dinner with my cousin Phil and his wife, Caroline. They visited three days into the new ordeal. Until then, Mia hadn't shown any signs of paranoia or thought disorder, only a desperate and growing concern to sleep through the night. It all changed while they were with us.

Phil, funny and entertaining, was telling a childhood story about breaking down in his old car with a high school friend. He was using phrases like, "We couldn't get that car running to save our lives" and "We tried to jump it but that wasn't working." Caroline and I were following along and laughing, but my focus was on Mia. She was unable to find any humor in what he was saying. She didn't mention anything at the time; she only sat and observed like someone trying to understand a foreign movie.

When they left, and the kids were getting ready for bed, I confronted her. "What did you think of Phil's story?"

"Pat, I didn't understand it," she conceded, looking more confused than worried. "The car was broken down, why would that threaten their lives? And why would he and his friend want to jump over their car? It didn't make any sense."

Dr. Rojas, already on high alert, didn't wait any longer. We started the olanzapine and Ativan immediately, and poor Mia started down the same dreadful path. Handing her the pills that night was heart-wrenching, like not only watching that drowning victim but throwing the anchor that drags her under.

Mia was lost again to the overmedicated paranoia that had become her alter ego. I knew it would be weeks before we started to titrate the medication, and then we would head into months of living with the unhappy stranger. After that, we would witness a period of reemergence, the butterfly crawling out of its blackened chrysalis. Finally, the wonderful person that was my wife would reappear, and we would relish her presence for a few months. But then, like a monster slithering through the night, the illness would steal her away again.

She was stabilized by mid-October, turned once more into an emotionally blunted zombie. Back at work, I arranged a call with Dr. Rojas. I wanted to speak to him without Mia overhearing.

After providing a quick update on her condition, I launched into a necessary but unpleasant conversation. "Dr. Rojas," I said, probably more forcefully than intended, "can you and I agree that this is not a onetime event?"

Silence. I continued, "Look, I want to start this conversation by telling you how much I respect your expertise and value your partnership. You have been the greatest support to Mia and me over the past two years. And so please know that I am not passing judgment on you as a psychiatrist."

"I know you aren't, Pat," he responded softly.

"Good, because we need you now more than ever. But this approach is not working."

"I agree. The pattern is becoming clear."

"Right." I was thankful that he wasn't clinging to his prior prognosis. "We need to figure this out for Mia and for the kids. She's missing life. I can't bear to watch it. And the whiplash is impossible for us." My voice was breaking, tears beginning to form.

"I know," he said in his calm and measured way, "but Pat, I have never seen anything like this."

"Alright," I said, gaining my composure, "but we have to ask ourselves the question, don't we? Is this schizophrenia?"

Dr. Rojas didn't hesitate. "Mia asked me that before, and you heard my answer. Schizophrenia doesn't fit."

"So, what is it? We need to find an answer!" I was raising my voice without realizing it, like if I demanded it loud enough, the solution might miraculously pop into his head.

"I have been through the *DSM* over and over again," he said. "I have spoken to colleagues, conducted my own research. I do not have an answer for you." He had referenced the *DSM*, that holy grail for psychiatrists. I had pored through the manual myself for years, all to no avail.

I wasn't mad at Dr. Rojas, but I was beyond frustrated. In a steady list of psychiatrists, he was the one I trusted most. He had become more than a doctor; he was a friend. He had been with us the longest and had observed Mia through every phase of her trial. If he had reached a dead end, where could we go next?

"Dr. Rojas, there must be something we are missing," I pleaded.

"You're right," he said, "but I can't identify it. Believe me, Pat, if I had any thoughts, I would be sharing them."

All I could see was Mia's sedated face from that morning, her deadened eyes devoid of life. I couldn't accept it; I couldn't give up on her. A sudden idea struck me.

"Dr. Rojas," I said, "if this were your wife, the person you loved most in the world, what would you do?"

He didn't respond for a few moments. I could almost hear him thinking through the question on the other end of the line. "McLean," he said finally. "I'd take her to McLean."

"Okay, McLean it is," I said, grasping at the confidence in his voice. After a slight pause, I felt silly asking, "What is McLean, exactly?"

"McLean is the mental health hospital affiliated with Harvard, up in Boston. It's the best in the world. Find someone there who can see her, Pat. This is beyond my experience."

"Great," I said, feeling suddenly optimistic. "That's exactly what we'll do. But you're with me on this, right? You'll help?"

"Of course, anything you two need."

I hung up with a new sense of hope. Even as the illness ravaged our lives for a third time, we had a new path to follow. I needed to believe a solution could be found; Mia needed me to believe it. And now we would be returning yet again to the place where everything had started.

Harvard had introduced us. Maybe it could save us, too.

19.

THE FINAL DIAGNOSIS

Bob Dylan
"Shelter from the Storm"
0:10–0:27

I was fired five months into my role at the investment firm in Sarasota. I wish that I had walked away of my own volition, but I didn't.

I hadn't failed at much before, and certainly not at a job. I was the employee whom people loved, the one they wanted to replicate. I created more value for companies than what they paid me. Firing me was a bad business decision, I always made sure of that. At least, I thought I did.

Although I was shocked while it was happening, I quickly discovered that my termination coincided with the firing of about half the staff. The firm, which I had assumed was healthy and profitable, was actually losing money fast. They had to cut salaries in an attempt to survive. Again, I derided myself for not having done more research on the business beforehand.

Thanks to our sale of internet stock, Mia and I could survive without the income for a while. At nights and on the weekends, I had been developing a few startup ideas. If one of them gained traction, I could slip smoothly into a new position at a company of my own.

Nevertheless, the fact that I was fired was a devastating blow. It threw me into an unusual funk. Naturally optimistic and happy, I became worried and disillusioned.

As the days turned into weeks, I found that not receiving a salary was crippling my self-esteem. Although we had money tucked away, a regular paycheck gave me comfort that I was providing for Mia and the kids. It proved that my hard work was worth something; it proved that I was worth something.

I tried to act confident around the family, pretending to be my normal upbeat self, but Mia knew me too well. Even though she didn't make a big deal of it, she could tell that I was struggling.

One of my startups required overnight travel to New York City. Not only was I not being paid, but I was shelling out money to cover expenses. I felt guilty every time I went, like I was betraying the family's trust. My faith was wavering; I was second-guessing my decisions. *Was this trip really necessary?* I asked myself as I checked into the hotel again.

I unzipped my overnight bag and noticed a little note on top of my clothes. The handwriting was Mia's:

I love you now more than I ever have.

That was all it said, those nine words. But the weight behind them was extraordinary. By the way she had phrased it, I knew that she believed in me. She was proud that I was betting on myself, trying to make it happen for us.

It was a powerful and much-needed reminder—it didn't matter if I was fired. It didn't matter if any of my startup plans panned out. What mattered was that Mia and I had found each other and that we loved each other.

Knowing she had my back during those challenging times meant everything.

***

Shortly after my call with Dr. Rojas, I ran an internet search on McLean Hospital. Although it was affiliated with Harvard Medical School, it wasn't located near the main Harvard campus. No wonder I wasn't familiar with it. But the institution had been around for almost two hundred years, and it was known as one of the leading mental health centers in the world.

The McLean website offered pages on each of the major mental illnesses, and I found myself returning to the section on bipolar and schizophrenia. Both involved psychosis, and both had been discussed with Mia's psychiatrists in the past.

I was already familiar with these diseases, although I knew more about bipolar than schizophrenia. The more I read about schizophrenia on the website, the more concerned I grew. Dr. Rojas was adamant that Mia didn't suffer from it, but the McLean information had me second-guessing his conclusion. She had periodic bouts of psychotic thought disorder, that was for sure. And during an episode, she was quick to slip into paranoid delusions. Maybe she had a strange form of schizophrenia with only some of the symptoms?

Bipolar was far more common and sounded easier to manage. McLean offered several treatment options for both, including short- and long-term care programs. They were all pricey, even the shorter ones; they ran over $25,000 per week. I tried to put that out of my mind. I would focus on finding a solution and then worry about how to afford it.

My bigger concern was the voluntary nature of the programs. By this point, Mia probably would agree to a residential facility as long as it didn't take her away from the kids for too long. But if she suffered a relapse during the program, she would definitely leave. Hopefully, McLean had solutions to deal with such contingencies.

I dialed the toll-free number listed on the page for bipolar and schizophrenia. A friendly woman answered, and I summarized our situation as succinctly as possible. She asked many questions about exact symptoms and medications. She found it telling that we had met with several psychiatrists, none of whom suggested schizophrenia as a diagnosis.

"One of the doctors," she asked, "did mention bipolar as a potential cause, is that correct?"

"That is correct. Dr. Martinez, who spent time with Mia in the crisis center, thought that she showed signs of mania."

"But she has never shown signs of depression?"

"Well, she did when she was taking the Prozac."

"Right, you did say that." The woman paused. I was impressed with McLean already. I wasn't sure if the person on the phone was a medical practitioner, but she was certainly investing the time to understand Mia's illness in detail. "But at this time, with your current psychiatrist, you remain unsure about the proper diagnosis?"

"Yes. Dr. Rojas and I are looking for someone at McLean to offer another perspective."

"Sir," she said, as if she had reached a sudden conclusion, "you need to speak with someone at the Pavilion, McLean's comprehensive diagnostic center. That's where we direct patients whose symptoms do not tell a clear story. The practitioners there have seen all kinds of cases."

A few moments later, I was talking with a woman named Cathy McCool. She cheerfully introduced herself as the director of admissions at the Pavilion. After about fifteen minutes of collecting information from me, she began telling me more about the center.

"For the most part, the Pavilion is a two-week residential treatment program. We are also self-pay, meaning that we will not accept insurance."

"That's okay," I said. "I don't think our insurance would cover it, anyway."

"That's unfortunate. Many patients are able to receive reimbursement from their insurance carriers. It is possible that the doctor will agree to consult with your current psychiatrist on an outpatient basis. That has happened before."

"I want to do whatever will help my wife get better. If it means residential treatment, we'll figure out how to afford it."

"I understand, Mr. Dylan. To be clear, Dr. Vuckovic has to agree to take the case."

"Oh?" I was surprised. "I thought as long as we agreed to the fee, we could be seen."

"No, it doesn't work that way," she explained. "Dr. Vuckovic will only accept patients whom he believes he can help. You will need to send copies of all medical records pertaining to your wife's illness, including your initial visit to the emergency room in Melbourne. Also, your current psychiatrist should provide a summary of your wife's case in as much detail as possible."

"Okay," I said. Gathering all the materials would take some effort. "May I ask, though, what percent of cases does he accept?"

"I'm not sure I could answer that accurately. But if he thinks he can help, he will see your wife. Once we have received the information, you should hear back from him within two weeks."

I hung up feeling hopeful and quickly googled Dr. Vuckovic. He was the medical director at the Pavilion and had been in that position for over ten years. He had spent his entire career working in mental health, most of it at McLean. He had a degree from Harvard Medical School, where he maintained a part-time appointment in the psychiatry department.

At that moment, I decided that Mia would see Dr. Vuckovic. I would do whatever it took—I wouldn't stop until she met with him.

Dr. Rojas was my first call, and he echoed my excitement. He promised to begin working on his write-up immediately. I then started the long process of requesting medical records. It was easier to have them faxed directly to the Pavilion, but I wanted copies, too. This meant that additional forms had to be completed. The whole affair took weeks, given that Mia and I had seen so many doctors when she was sick, including not only multiple psychiatrists but emergency room doctors, primary care physicians, neurologists, gynecologists, and other specialists.

Finally, by the end of October, I had collected the last of Mia's medical records and sent them off to McLean. I also received a copy of Dr. Rojas's letter, which he sent directly to the Pavilion. After sending an email to Cathy, confirming that all materials had been delivered, I began waiting for Dr. Vuckovic's answer.

It was impossible to guess the odds that he would take Mia's case. I still didn't know much about McLean, and I had never spoken to him directly. Cathy was as affable and helpful as possible, but what mattered was Dr. Vuckovic's expertise. I bided my time, thinking up strategies for dealing with rejection.

Fortunately, these weren't necessary. About a week later, Cathy called to share the good news that our case had been accepted, and the even better news that Dr. Vuckovic was willing to meet with Mia on an outpatient basis. In a long sequence of bad breaks, we finally had something to celebrate.

I still hadn't broached the idea of going to McLean with Mia. On the phone with Cathy, I had scheduled our visit for early December; it was the closest date available on Dr. Vuckovic's calendar. But Mia remained on heavy doses of olanzapine, and I wasn't sure how she would react. Resisting the temptation to delay the discussion, I sat down with her that evening.

Rather than become upset, Mia responded positively. She was grateful that I had gone to the trouble of arranging the visit and, after reviewing the website and Dr. Vuckovic's background, impressed with the Pavilion's resources. She wasn't enthusiastic, but I didn't expect her to be. She was on too much medication to show excitement.

But I was ecstatic. I wrote my own letter to Dr. Vuckovic, thanking him for taking Mia's case and providing my perspective of her disease. I focused on summarizing the pattern of the illness as I saw it. Hopefully, the more information he had, the more likely he could accurately diagnose the problem.

On an afternoon in early December, we caught a flight up to Boston. We were in the midst of titrating the olanzapine, but Dr. Rojas and I had agreed not to make any changes to the dose during the days leading up to our trip. Mia lacked energy but her personality was stable.

I had booked a hotel right on the Charles River, close to Harvard's campus. You could see the red dome of Dunster House silhouetted against the bridges spanning the water. The weather was frigid that night, but I felt warm in the rich memories of the time that we had spent together in Cambridge.

Our appointment wasn't until after lunch. McLean was a half-hour drive, and we arrived on the campus just before noon. It looked more like a collection of old houses and buildings than a hospital. Set back among barren trees in the dead of winter, the snowy fields probably became tranquil lawns of grass in the spring and summer. I was reminded of a well-endowed preparatory school.

We parked near the Wyman Building, where the Pavilion was located, and tracked through the cold to the central cafeteria. After a quiet lunch, we entered the front doors of the Wyman Building, a two-story brick mansion with white colonnades on the porch. Inside, the house was ancient but well maintained, with dark wood floors and intricate crown molding. The furniture and rugs were old, but the place had a quiet air of dignity. It reminded me of many of Harvard's timeworn buildings.

Cathy, her kind smile reflecting the friendly voice with which I had become familiar, ushered us into a small waiting room on the second floor. We sat on wooden chairs, listening intently for voices leaking from the surrounding offices.

Soon, one of the doors opened and Dr. Vuckovic stepped out. I recognized him immediately, with his gray hair parted to the side and intelligent-looking glasses. He was wearing a dark suit and tie, and a serious but pleasant smile flashed across his face. "Mia?" he asked, and we stood up. "It is a pleasure to meet you." He offered her an outstretched hand. "And you must be Pat?"

"Yes, sir," I said, shaking his hand in turn. "Thank you so much for seeing us."

"It's my pleasure. I'd like to meet with Mia alone at first, if that's okay with both of you?"

I looked at Mia, hoping that she wouldn't be put off. Thankfully, she didn't seem fazed. "Yes, of course," I said.

"Thank you. I'd like you to join us in a while. If you could just wait here?"

"Sure."

He led Mia into his office and shut the door behind them.

In the silence of that old house that reminded me so much of college, I began reminiscing about how Mia and I had met, about those early years: hearing George beg her for pizza on a Saturday night; catching sight of her dancing across the room at my house formal; seeing her face light up with a surprised smile when I began my wedding toast in Spanish; watching her read a storybook aloud in our new Florida home, our small children snuggled on her lap.

But then those memories faded, replaced abruptly by different ones: Mia rambling incoherently about prison in the pitch dark of morning; berating a kindhearted nun for standing in a Sunday school classroom; battling the door of our lanai in a frantic attempt to escape; whipping confetti-torn pictures at me with malice etched across her face; crying uncontrollably on our front porch surrounded by first responders, red lights flashing in the background.

I snapped out of my ruminating and glanced around the room. How many other people had waited in my same chair, thinking about how their lives had been shattered by mental illness? Had the Pavilion been able to solve their mysteries, or did they still live with the devastation wreaked by their diseases? I could hear people on the first floor, the upbeat voice of Cathy greeting someone at the front door. It was a normal day at McLean; Mia was just another patient in a long line of suffering.

As much as I tried, I couldn't hear what Dr. Vuckovic and Mia were discussing. What questions were being asked—the same ones that had been posed a thousand times already? I hoped that she was answering them truthfully, opening up to him the way she did to me. More than anything, I hoped he was uncovering some clue that had been overlooked, some insight that might unlock an answer.

After what seemed like an hour, Dr. Vuckovic opened the door. "Pat, would you care to join us now?"

I walked into his office, with its many bookcases and its large mahogany desk. Mia was seated in front of it, and

I took my place in the chair next to her. He sat opposite us. Her medical records were spread out before him.

"I wanted to thank you for your letter, Pat," Dr. Vuckovic started. "It was incredibly helpful."

"Thank you," I said, pleasantly surprised.

"As you noted, there seems to be a clear pattern associated with Mia's condition."

"That's right." I took Mia's hand. She was watching Dr. Vuckovic with interest.

"I have been the head of this diagnostic center for the past eleven years," Dr. Vuckovic said. "During that time, I have seen well over a thousand cases, all fairly complicated. Prior to my time here, I saw thousands more." He paused to look up over his glasses. "I am, I fear, older than you two."

Smiling, he glanced down at Mia's file again. "All in all, I have probably seen five thousand patients in my career, maybe more. And in all that time, I have seen exactly three that I believe share a condition with Mia."

I caught my breath. "Three people?"

"Yes, three people. And interestingly enough, two of them were related. A brother and a sister." He sat back in his chair. "Mia, I believe that you are suffering from unipolar mania."

She didn't react.

"Unipolar mania?" I asked. "I've never heard of that. It isn't in the *DSM*."

He smiled and chuckled. "Impressive," he said. "You've done your homework, Pat. But not everything is in the *DSM*. Like I said, I have seen this only three times before. It is not only rare; it is exceedingly rare."

"Dr. Vuckovic," Mia interrupted. "What is it? Is it treatable?" Her voice startled me; I hadn't expected her to say anything.

He turned to her. "Unipolar mania is related to bipolar, Mia, except without the depression. Most people would prefer to experience only the manic phase. It gives you more energy, makes you feel invincible; and, as you know all too well, it requires far fewer hours of sleep. But at its most extreme, and left untreated, mania can lead to psychosis.

"That's what I believe is happening here. Everyone naturally goes through phases of feeling up and feeling down, controlled by various chemicals in our brains and throughout our bodies. We psychiatrists don't know as much about this as we'd like, unfortunately. We do know that for those with bipolar disorder, these phases are more extreme."

He stopped for a moment, apparently thinking about some of his patients, before continuing.

"They are more extreme and more problematic. When someone with bipolar goes through the down phase, they suffer depression. In some cases, their depression can become suicidal, and they become a threat to themselves. But the up phase, the manic phase, can also be dangerous. Sure, people might feel more productive and creative, but mania can become quite destructive. People take too many risks, spend their money in foolish gambles, or cheat on their loved ones. And, as I mentioned, it can turn psychotic." He paused again.

"I believe you suffer from a form of bipolar that doesn't include depression. Your condition manifests itself only with periodic mania. But, unfortunately, that mania leads quickly to psychotic mania."

Silence filled the room. It made complete sense to me. We had always been told that bipolar wasn't applicable because Mia had never suffered depression. But what if she didn't need to? Her behavior was manic at the outset, with the troubled sleep and heightened energy levels. And when she finally broke with reality, it took unbelievable amounts of medication to stop her brain from spinning.

Mia's face was a mixture of acceptance and fear. "Dr. Vuckovic," I said, weighing my words carefully, "if Mia does present symptoms of unipolar mania, what's the prognosis? There must be a way to treat this effectively."

He smiled slightly, nodding his head. "I do have some good news there. The challenge in treating bipolar is that the medication for one phase can swing a person to the other end of the spectrum. And psychotropic drugs affect people in different ways. Determining the optimal balance of medications for a specific individual can be quite difficult. But in your case, Mia, we only need moderate the manic phase. We need to keep you from spilling over into psychosis."

We were listening closely, hanging on to his every word. "Fortunately, we have a drug that does this quite effectively. It's called lithium. Lithium is actually a naturally occurring element that happens to be an excellent mood-stabilizing agent. It's one of those strange things in the world of mental health. We know that lithium works—we've been using it effectively for over fifty years—but we don't know why it works. All I can tell you is that I put the prior three patients with this condition on lithium, and they never suffered these symptoms again."

"Never again?" I asked eagerly. "That was it?"

"Well, I shouldn't say 'never again,' because I don't know for certain. But in the time during which they communicated with me, and it was many years, they never became psychotic again. I don't have a recent update, but I assume they have been fine, or we would have heard from them."

Mia was suddenly engaged, asking about the possible side effects and long-term consequences of lithium. She was the physician assistant, trying to learn as much as possible from an expert in the field, but I was only partially listening. My mind was reflecting on this new, seemingly miraculous, information.

Ever since my battle with Crohn's disease, I had been convinced that health problems weren't solved by seeing the right doctor and taking the right pill. They were addressed by lifestyle changes, eating the right foods, exercising regularly, and avoiding stress. But here at McLean, with this menacing disease that had caused so much suffering, I was hoping that Dr. Vuckovic would prove me wrong.

I did catch some of their conversation, which had turned more pragmatic. Lithium had few short-term consequences. It could lead to weight gain, like all the other psychiatric drugs seemed to do, and could also interfere with thyroid function. But these seemed rare and manageable. Over a longer period of time, lithium could cause permanent kidney damage. This was a more serious risk, but apparently, with careful monitoring it could be avoided.

They were then discussing a treatment plan. Mia would continue working with Dr. Rojas, who would oversee her care, with Dr. Vuckovic consulting as needed. She could start on lithium as soon as she weaned off olanzapine.

Watching Mia, I thought she looked unconvinced. She would try lithium because we were desperate. But we had tried Prozac, too, and that didn't end well.

Nonetheless, McLean gave me confidence. I was impressed by Dr. Vuckovic. His diagnosis was the most plausible I had heard, and he had successfully treated patients who had exhibited similar symptoms.

On the way back to the airport, Mia and I rehashed our conversation with Dr. Vuckovic and speculated about unipolar mania. She was more upbeat than I anticipated. We called Dr. Rojas once we were through security, and he was fascinated. Although surprised, he put his faith in McLean and was looking forward to working with Dr. Vuckovic.

As we took off over the buildings of Boston, I felt my spirits rising along with the plane. After almost two and a half years of suffering, could we finally put the past behind us? If so, Mia and I could repair the life that we had built together.

I thought that if we could restore Mia's health, the rest would be easy.

20.

THE CHRISTMAS PRESENT

Foo Fighters
"Walk"
0:38–1:06

Our first couple of years in Florida were hard for me. Mia had dedicated herself full-time to raising the kids, which we both felt was important. She was planning to work again in a few years, while I was desperately trying to earn a living after becoming unemployed.

Given my past success as an entrepreneur, I assumed that starting a company would be the solution, but it was slow going. Neither Mia nor I came from wealth, and watching our savings dwindle with every bill was demoralizing.

I used to stop at a gas station around the corner from our house. As I was pumping, I couldn't help but notice the huge, colorful sign in the window of the convenience store: "Florida Lotto" it read, in bright green and white. It always showed the current prize amount, which usually exceeded $10 million. I knew better than to play, but that sign taunted me—the guy without a real job, the guy who couldn't provide for his family.

After putting the kids to bed one night, Mia and I began talking about the future. It had been almost two years since we had moved down from Boston. Although she loved living in Florida, Mia was fully supportive of relocating if it wasn't going to work.

"I don't know," I complained, disappointed that I hadn't been able to gain more traction. "I like it here, but it feels like I'm not getting anywhere."

"Then let's move back," she said. "It's not worth it if you aren't happy."

"I'm happy. It's just that, well, I can't fool around forever. We've already spent everything we earmarked for this adventure."

"Okay, then we move."

I shook my head. I knew that she meant it, but I also knew that she loved the warm weather. And we both treasured being close to our families. "It shouldn't be this hard," I said, more to myself than anything. "I should be able to figure this out."

"Maybe we sell the house?" she suggested. "At least that way we wouldn't be tied down. It would give us more flexibility."

"No, if we sold the house, we'd definitely move."

"Then I don't know what we're talking about this for. It's pretty clear that we should just go."

She was probably right, but I didn't want to admit defeat. Leaving would feel like surrender. If only we had more time. Suddenly, the image of that Lotto sign popped into my head. More money would give us more time.

"I wish I could just win the lottery," I mumbled.

"What?"

"I said, 'I wish I could win the lottery,'" I answered a bit louder.

Mia took a moment to reply. "Pat," she said, "you already have."

She waited, giving her words even more impact. "You were born into a supportive family in a free country. You were blessed with intelligence and ambition. You attended one of the most elite universities in the world—twice." Her unblinking eyes observed me sternly. "And you're white." A second pause. "And you're a man."

It was a profound rebuke, made all the more powerful by its truth.

"What more do you want?" she finished sharply.

I was speechless. She was right, of course. I had nothing to complain about. It was the single greatest thing anyone has ever said to me. And I have carried it with me every day since, especially during the troubled times that have been recounted in this story.

After that, I went out of my way to stop at that particular gas station. And every time I looked at that sign, it filled me with gratitude. Because Mia had nailed it: when it came to life, I had already hit the jackpot.

***

Three months into the new year, after having fully weaned her from the olanzapine, Dr. Rojas started Mia on lithium. We began the new medication gradually, warily looking for any side effects. Fortunately, she adapted well to it, and within a few weeks all concerns had dissipated. Soon, her former personality began to resurface. By the beginning of summer, our house once again returned to its previous state, filled with liveliness and harmony.

These were easier months for Mia and me, in terms of managing her health. Once the lithium didn't show any adverse consequences, we could relax a bit. We both knew that the disease provided periods of recovery; we didn't expect another relapse for at least six months. And while we continued to monitor her sleep carefully, she had reverted to old patterns. She fell asleep easily and slept at least eight hours every night.

In August, the kids started classes. Will was beginning high school, and Jamie was in seventh grade. Maybe it was the heightened level of activity, or the anxiety that came with the start of the academic year, but the past three falls had seemed to increase Mia's vulnerability. September and October had been difficult months for us.

I was steadfastly looking out for any signs of trouble. In early September, I noticed that Mia was more energetic than usual. Although she was sleeping fine at night, she was hustling around with a huge list of priorities during the day. I mentioned it after dinner a couple of nights into her high-octane schedule. Will remained at the table doing homework.

"Babe, have you noticed that you have more energy than usual?" I asked.

Without stopping whatever she was doing in the kitchen, she replied, "No, I don't think so, but I do need to get this done by tomorrow."

Will looked up from his book. He gave me a slight smile and said, "Mom, you should listen to Dad. I've noticed it, too."

Mia immediately stopped and walked over, her eyes wide. "Really?" she asked.

"Yeah," he replied, nodding his head.

"Okay, I'll call Dr. Rojas first thing tomorrow."

Dr. Rojas increased her lithium dosage immediately, and a remarkable thing happened: the illness didn't progress. Within a couple of weeks, she no longer felt such high energy. In fact, she found herself becoming lethargic and sleeping in later.

It was an immense triumph for us. Clearly, the higher exposure to lithium helped her body defend itself from another relapse. Although not ready to declare victory, we became cautiously more optimistic.

The other positive result was that Mia took over the relationship with Dr. Rojas. In years prior, given that she was periodically so sick, I had been forced to take the lead. But once they could rely on the medication to maintain her health, Mia and Dr. Rojas learned together how to manage her lithium dosage more effectively. Dr. Vuckovic was available for counsel, but they didn't need much of his input. He provided the kernel of advice, and then Mia and Dr. Rojas became experts themselves.

Knowing the potential long-term effects on her kidneys, Mia began a schedule of having blood tests performed on a regular basis. She and Dr. Rojas would then carefully review the results, monitoring her body's lithium levels. But more than anything, they would rely on Mia's own evaluation of her mood. Over time, she began to realize how much energy was too much.

Given that the crisis had been averted, our family enjoyed its first holiday season in years. We felt whole again, with Mia joining the festivities. As the new year started, and the illness receded more distantly into the past, new memories with the kids began to replace unfortunate moments from prior years.

That summer, I planned a ten-day family vacation that involved renting a car and driving through the English countryside, stopping at small towns, staying at B&Bs, and taking hikes together. I wanted us to be close physically, hoping it might help to recapture the emotional warmth that had characterized our family before.

One night, we were gathered at a crowded restaurant where the locals were encouraged to bring their pets along. As I was walking back to our table from the restroom, I noticed Mia and the kids watching me and giggling.

"Okay, what's the joke?" I asked, a smile now stretching across my face, too.

"It looks like someone's in love with you, Pat," said Mia, nodding her head toward the far corner. When I glanced over, I saw the cutest King Charles spaniel, its eyes glued to me. I stood up, walked back the way I had come, and then retraced my steps to our table. The dog's intense stare followed my every move.

As I sat back down, Jamie quipped, "Yeah, I think that dog wants to marry you!"

I immediately looked to Mia. Instinctively, I was worried that she might take Jamie's comment literally. But Mia didn't miss a beat. "That's fine with me," she said. "Then that dog will be the one dealing with Dad's bad breath in the morning!"

The kids howled, and I couldn't help but laugh myself. Our old Mia was back, and she was thriving. Without the whiplash of ongoing relapses, her relationship with the kids was as strong as ever.

Indeed, everything was going great. Will and Jamie were growing up; and, although going through the normal challenges of adolescence, they were flourishing. Scars from Mia's illness had healed. It didn't appear that the kids would suffer any lasting effects from the experience. And Mia's confidence was growing with every month of continued health. Her generous and supportive personality was fully restored, along with her sense of humor. Coming home to a house full of happy and positive people became my daily highlight.

After a year on the lithium with no relapses, Mia and I were enthusiastic. After two years, we were confident in its efficacy. And the years were flying by, as they do when you have two teenagers in the house. By all accounts, our war with the illness was over. Everyone seemed to have moved on, putting the conflict behind them. Everyone, that is, except me.

I suffered recurring nightmares—a lot of them. They ran through similar themes. Mia and I would be locked in our room, and she would be fully psychotic. She would be screaming about going in reverse or quietly revealing a secret theory to me, and my adrenaline would skyrocket. The spooky eeriness of psychosis would overwhelm me, and I'd wake up in a pool of sweat with my heart racing.

Other times, I would dream I was in a dark room. I couldn't touch them, but I knew that Mia and the kids were nearby. And suddenly a sinister force would begin circling outside, searching for a way in. Protecting them was all that mattered to me, but I couldn't figure out how to keep them safe. I couldn't see anything, but I sensed the monster close at hand. Usually, I would wake myself up by screaming at it, an actual shout echoing in our bedroom. I'd frequently wake Mia up, too.

Although disturbing, I didn't think such dreams were unusual. I had been through a lot, and my brain was still trying to process the ordeal. If it meant dealing with terrors at night, so be it. At least Mia and the kids were safe and healthy in real life.

But other problems continued to plague me. I couldn't walk through our house without scenes from the ordeal flashing through my mind: our bedroom with all of its psychotic memories, the dinner table with its many uncomfortable conversations, the back room where Luke had wrestled Mia to the floor. The worst was the front porch, where I had watched my wife being handcuffed and taken away; I tried to avoid it.

In addition, the defenses I had constructed against being hurt again remained fully in place, and I still treated Mia like a friend rather than a spouse. I kept telling myself that time would mend the wounds of the past; if I just gave things enough time, the intimacy between us would reestablish itself.

Except that it didn't. Finally, after nearly four years, Mia came to me one night in our room.

"Pat, we need to talk," she said, not with malice but with sincere empathy in her voice. I knew immediately what it was about.

"Okay." I was unsure how to react.

"What are we doing? Who are we anymore?"

I sat looking at her without the ability to respond.

"I know things were really hard on you when I was sick, and I can't thank you enough for everything you did for me." Her eyes began to water. "Without you, I don't know what would have happened to me."

I was becoming emotional, too. We didn't talk much about her illness. It was too hard on both of us.

"And so, I'll be forever grateful to you." She sniffed a bit, and then laughed, her breath releasing in a small gasp. "I don't know what I ever did to deserve someone like you."

I still hadn't spoken. I knew what she was going to say, and I wasn't ready for it.

"But I don't know what we are doing. Are we just friends now? Is that all we're going to be?"

"I don't know. No, that's not what I meant," I quickly corrected myself. "That's not all we're going to be."

"Are you waiting for the kids to graduate, and then you'll ask for a divorce?"

"No, Mia, no. That's not what I want at all!" At that moment, I realized the dire consequences of my neglect. I had fought with all my strength for this woman, for our future, and I had won. But here I was, on the brink of losing everything.

My brain wasn't capable of reacting. It was like I was standing behind those defenses, trying to peer over them to see Mia again—the Mia I had fallen in love with. But I couldn't get myself to jump over the barrier.

Her expression softened. "Pat, you need to get help."

"What do you mean?"

She smiled gently and put her hand on mine. "You made sure everyone had support when I was sick—everyone except for you."

"I had Luke, he was there with me."

"Yeah, Luke was great, but that's not what I'm talking about. You need to see a therapist. You have real issues, and you need to deal with them."

My first reaction was denial. I was the strong one, the one who had saved the family. I had dealt with the illness; I could deal with anything. "I just need more time," I said.

"You've had almost four years. That's a lot of time."

Her words hit home. "You're right," I said. And that was how we left it. I didn't commit to anything, but she had made a strong argument. More importantly, she had planted the thought in my head. And the more I pondered it, the more obvious it became. It was hard to believe that I hadn't seen it for myself.

The next day, I began reviewing profiles of psychologists. I had to be selective; our story was an agonizing one, and I didn't want to revisit it more than once. The search process took several days; investing a lot up front would hopefully improve my chances of finding a good match.

I kept coming back to one candidate. His name was Dr. Tomasz Nowak. He had a doctorate in clinical psychology and several other degrees, but that wasn't what caught my attention. What fascinated me were all the newspaper articles about him. He had been a Catholic priest in California but had relocated to Florida to establish his counseling practice after some kind of scandal. The Church claimed that he had misappropriated funds. They defrocked him, dragging his name through the papers while doing so.

But that stood in stark contrast to what his parishioners thought of him. I read one testimonial after another in which people claimed that Dr. Nowak was the most honest, most thoughtful person in the world. In fact, his congregation held a public rally as a last-ditch effort to keep him from being ousted. The more I read, the more it appeared that he had been the target of a jealous and vindictive bishop.

His ordeal mimicked my own. He had dedicated his life to a relationship, one with the Catholic Church, and then it had suddenly been stripped away. I wondered how he had dealt with that.

Soon, I was checking in at Dr. Nowak's office for my introductory session. I smiled inwardly as I walked into his lobby. The white noise was playing in the background, and the elegant couch sat under soothing pictures of tranquil landscapes. It felt strangely familiar but also very different. This time, I would be the one answering the questions.

When he greeted me, I knew immediately that he was not the villain the Church had made him out to be. He had a warm smile and kind eyes, and his Polish accent embellished a voice that was at once generous and trustworthy. My gut told me that he was the correct choice. Dr. Nowak, or "Dr. Tom" as he insisted, was the right person to help me pick through the rubble of the past.

Most of the first session was a steady stream of storytelling. Dr. Tom posed questions now and again, but he mostly listened. Near the end of our time together, he asked, "You have focused a lot of the story on how it impacted Mia and your children, but have you thought about its effect on you?"

"Yes, I have, more since Mia and I talked about it."

"And?"

"And I don't think that I'll ever feel as close to anyone as I felt with Mia before she got sick. But that was a kind of naïve closeness, the closeness of someone too young to understand that life can be so harsh. You can't let yourself feel that connected to anybody. You can't really ever know what someone else is thinking, that has become obvious to me. And then, if you do have a relationship like that, and you lose it, it's just too painful. It's like losing a loved one."

"Do you feel like you lost Mia?" he asked.

"No, I don't feel like I lost Mia. She's the same person she was before." I realized that he had made his point. "But I lost her for a while," I added quickly, "and I didn't know if I would ever get her back."

Dr. Tom ended our appointment saying he thought he could help. For me, the experience was surprisingly cathartic. Up to that point, I hadn't spoken much about Mia's illness to anyone. Our family members and close friends knew it had been difficult, but they didn't know the details. Luke knew some of them; he had lived through the worst with me. But just talking to Dr. Tom about what had happened helped me feel better.

Although we didn't discuss his background, he knew the reason I had chosen him. We felt a kinship, and it made it easier for me to open up. I agreed that we should work together, and we scheduled a set of recurring weekly meetings.

My first appointment with Dr. Tom was right around the holidays, and I prepared a special card for Mia. After the Christmas Day festivities were concluded, I pulled her aside in our bedroom.

"This is my actual present to you, babe," I said, handing her the envelope. Inside, I had included Dr. Tom's business card, with a note that I was taking her recommendation seriously.

"Pat," she replied, those familiar eyes pulling me in, "I can't tell you how much this means to me." She wrapped me in a hug, resting her head against my shoulder. "It might be hard, but I'll support you any way I can."

I quickly discovered that Mia was right, the next steps were not going to be easy. In subsequent meetings, Dr. Tom began probing into the worst parts of our ordeal. Several times, he made me relive the actual experience, describing to him in detail a specific scene and how it made me feel. I told him about the terror of the first day and the exhaustion of the first week. I recounted the Plan and the Devil and the battles of the crisis center.

Every time we met, my body's fight-or-flight response would trigger, with my heartbeat soaring and my palms sweating, even though we were sitting in the peaceful serenity of Dr. Tom's office. The worst session was when we replayed the night of the 911 call.

Several weeks into our relationship, he made a startling announcement. "Pat, I believe that you suffer from post-traumatic stress disorder. It is typically referred to as PTSD."

I laughed. "I've heard of PTSD, but that affects soldiers coming home from war. What we went through was tough, and sometimes I refer to it as a battle, but it was nothing like that."

"It's true that many soldiers suffer PTSD," Dr. Tom explained, "but you don't need to have experienced a combat situation. Any traumatic event or experience can lead to PTSD, and you fit that description."

"Look, I agree that we went through some difficult times, but it didn't lead to my own mental illness." I was the rock, the solid foundation for our family. Sure, I needed some help, but I wasn't in the midst of a crisis. "It isn't affecting my life," I said.

"Really?" Dr. Tom asked. "*I don't think that I'll ever feel as close to anyone as I felt with Mia before she got sick,*" he said, quoting me. "One of the revealing characteristics of PTSD is an inability to develop and maintain close relationships, a loss of hope about returning to a normal life."

"Yeah, but—"

"And another symptom: trying to avoid thinking or talking about the event that caused the trauma. If Mia hadn't prodded you, and we hadn't met, would you have ever revisited what happened?"

"Well, maybe not, but—"

"And another one: recurring nightmares related to the event. Sound familiar?"

"Right, but—"

"Pat, listen to yourself. You and I both know that mental illness is real. Why are you pushing back so hard on this?"

I stopped protesting. He was right. The experience had impacted me more than I was willing to admit. I admired Mia for recognizing her challenge and rising to it, adopting the behaviors that would lead to recovery. It was time for me to step up, for her sake and mine.

We spent the rest of our session talking about PTSD, including its symptoms and the prognosis. I was fortunate; treatment didn't always require strong medications. In some cases, simply talking could provide tremendous benefits, as I had already found.

"Dr. Tom, is there anything I can do on my own, when I'm not here with you?"

"I do have one suggestion, Pat," he said, "but it won't be easy."

"What is it?"

"Write," he replied. "Write it all down. Everything."

"You mean, write it down like in a book or something?"

"In whatever way you want. By writing it down you'll relive it, and in reliving it you'll continue your process of healing. You'll take control of what happened."

It was an interesting concept, one that I wouldn't have considered on my own, but I remained skeptical. Talking with Dr. Tom about the illness was hard enough; I didn't welcome the thought of revisiting the details again.

But I kept coming back to the idea. It wouldn't cost me anything, and if it didn't help, I could always stop. Plus, I could do it in secret; no one else would need to know. If I truly wanted to heal—to recoup what Mia and I had lost—I should be open to anything. I owed it to us; I owed it to our family.

Thinking about the family led me back to my mom's advice to make sure the kids felt safe, wanted, and loved. Suddenly, I realized how accurately it applied to our experience with mental illness.

In the beginning, my focus was on keeping Mia safe. Although she didn't like the crisis center, I knew it would protect her. And Luke, with his warm and wild personality, kept everyone feeling more secure, especially Mia. Then, during the long periods of recovery, I struggled to make her feel wanted, even though, with her changed personality, life was easier when she wasn't in the room.

Now, over six years later, we were beyond all of that. It was time for the final step. I never stopped loving Mia, but she couldn't feel it anymore. And no wonder: the closeness that had defined our relationship was gone. My own illness was blocking the final phase of our healing.

I had to accept my disease and recognize its challenges. I had to feel safe, wanted, and loved, too. *Deep down, do I even feel safe?* I wondered. *I can't even walk through the house without thinking about what happened.*

That weekend, when I found myself alone for a few hours, I pulled out my laptop. I was sitting in the back room, gathering my strength to face the ghosts of prior years. Looking around, I could hear the echoes of a fierce struggle and the faint sirens of a night long past.

Turning on my computer, I imagined the guest bedroom of my parents' house on a Sunday morning in late September. Pitch black. Too quiet. An ominous feeling builds.

I hear my wife's voice in the darkness.

"Pat, I am going to prison," I typed, tears forming with the weight of the memory. I wiped my eyes, took a deep breath, and kept writing.

EPILOGUE

Queen and David Bowie
"Under Pressure"
2:37–3:32

Thankfully, Mia and I remain happily married. Dr. Tom helped me recognize and then overcome my own mental illness; writing this book was a crucial part of my recovery. The kids have since gone off to college, but that gives Mia and me more time to concentrate on each other. We are as close now as we have ever been.

But that's not her real name, and Patrick Dylan is not mine. I wanted to tell our story, but not everyone involved was supportive. Rather than disrupt relationships, I changed details—names, locations, et cetera. But events, dialogue, and emotions have been preserved. This is our story, even if you don't know who we are.

Shielding Mia from the stigma of mental illness was at the forefront of my mind when the ordeal began. It governed my actions and contributed greatly to my own stress during an already traumatic time. But a funny thing happened when people finally heard about her sickness: they began sharing their own experiences with us.

I was amazed by the number of friends who came forward. Anxiety and depression were common, and many admitted to taking medication either regularly or at some point in the past. Other serious conditions were also prevalent. One relative shared the story of her son's challenges with mental illness. One colleague revealed that his daughter suffered from bipolar disorder; another had a teen who was in and out of treatment centers. Still another close friend confided that for years he had struggled periodically with the very same symptoms that Mia had faced, including acute psychosis.

We never knew how many friends suffered in secret, but it shouldn't have been surprising; nearly 20 percent of Americans struggle with a mental illness. That means if you have ten friends, two of them are dealing with it right now. Do you know who they are? Probably not. Mental illness is something that we have been taught to hide.

The stigma has thousands of years behind it, built on a foundation of ignorance and fear. If someone started acting psychotic hundreds of years ago, people attributed it to demons, sorcery, or some other supernatural power. That person would have been locked away or put to death. No one understood that chemical imbalances in the brain were the root cause. Even something less extreme than psychosis would have been punished or ridiculed. And so, as a community, we learned to hide mental illness at all costs.

But now we know more. Psychiatrists have a better understanding of the neurotransmitters that control thought. We have plenty more to learn, but we know for certain that mental illness isn't "all in someone's head" or the result of evil spirits. Those concepts are foolish, but they still govern how we act toward it. As a result, too many people agonize in isolation, afraid to seek the help they so desperately need.

It doesn't have to be this way. As a society, we choose not to break the taboo around mental illness. We go along with the ridicule. We condone the behaviors that enforce the stigma. We hide our troubles away, hoping no one will learn the truth about the challenges we face.

We need to stop.

Every person in our family has been affected by mental illness. Why are we so ashamed to admit it? We wouldn't be embarrassed if heart disease lay at the center of this story; a disease of the brain shouldn't be any different. I look forward to a day when people can share their experiences with mental illness openly and honestly, without worrying about how the world will define them or upsetting the ones they love.

This is a story of strength, resilience, and hope. I wrote it as a dedication to the members of a special family, each of whom was crucial to our ultimate recovery. And I wrote it for my wife, who will always be the most special person in my life.

This is my story. I couldn't be prouder to tell it.

A NOTE FROM THE AUTHOR

Music has supported me through many difficult times, but it was never more important than during the events shared within these pages. I had intended that each chapter of this book begin with lyrics from the songs that formed the backdrop of this experience. I then learned that doing so would break dozens of copyright laws. Still, I felt an obligation to these artists. I listened to their songs nonstop during my struggle: in the car, on a run, in a dark room trying to find strength.

Although I couldn't include the lyrics, I have included the artist and title, as these are legal to print. If you'd like to know the particular words that were important to me, I've provided markers for those as well. Here's an example:

Talking Heads
"This Must Be the Place (Naïve Melody)"
2:49–3:22

And let me state this clearly to ward off any music-industry attorneys: *I am encouraging you to listen to this music!* This story definitely has a soundtrack, and I wanted to share it.

ACKNOWLEDGMENTS

A heartfelt thanks goes out to "Dr. Tom." Without your prompting, this book never would have been started. I send deep gratitude to Caroline and Pete, who read very early drafts and gave me the confidence and encouragement to continue. I would also like to thank other friends who provided feedback and support along the way, including Paul, Irene, Charlene, Jeanine, Chris, Beth, Julie, Angela, Dave, Joe, Deb, and Bill. The generous dedication of your time and advice improved the manuscript by leaps and bounds. All of the good people at Girl Friday Productions deserve the credit for making this book a reality, especially Katherine, Katie, and Laura. And, of course, I owe the world to my editors: the eagle-eyed Brittany, the incredibly talented Diana, and the always-amazing Jackie.

Thanks also to the many practitioners who provided care to us during this struggle, including John, Mike, Ronny, Eduardo, Jeremy, Jenny, Cathy, Alexander, and Stan. We will remain forever grateful for your advice and expertise.

Finally, to my wife and two kids: your support meant everything. Said more correctly, you mean everything. "If we can get through that, we can get through anything."

ABOUT THE AUTHOR

Patrick Dylan joins the voices calling for an end to the stigma surrounding mental illness. He and his wife, Mia, live in Florida and have two college-age children. They hope that sharing their family's story will spread awareness of the realities of mental illness and offer support to others who are either experiencing a mental health crisis or providing care to an affected loved one.

CPSIA information can be obtained
at www.ICGtesting.com
Printed in the USA
JSHW052103090322
23652JS00002B/119